Age	Physical Development	Social and Emotional Development	Intellectual Development	Language Development
At Birth	Lies in fetal position with knees tucked up. Unable to raise head. Head falls backwards if pulled to sit. Reacts to sudden sound. Closes eye to bright light. Opens eye when held in an upright position.	Bonds with mother. Smiles at mother.	Beginning to develop concepts e.g. becomes aware of physical sensations such as hunger. Explores using his senses. Make eye contact and cry to indicate need.	Cries vigorously. Respond to high-pitched tones by moving his limbs.
3 Months	Pelvis is flat when lying down. Lower back is still weak. Back and neck firm when held sitting. Grasps objects placed in hands. Turns head round to have a look at objects. Establishes eye contact.	Squeals with pleasure appropriately. Reacts with pleasure to familiar routines. Discriminates smile.	Takes increasing interest in his surroundings. Shows interest in playthings. Understand cause and effect... e.g. if you tie one end of a ribbon to his toe and the other to a mobile, he will learn to move the mobile.	Attentive to sounds made by your voice. Indicates needs with differentiated cries. Beginning to vocalise. Smile in response to speech.
6 Months	Can lift head and shoulders. Sits up with support. Enjoys standing and jumping. Transfers objects from one hand to the other. Pulls self up to sit and sits erect with supports. Rolls over prone to supine. Palmer grasp of cube. Well established visual sense.	Responds to different tones of mother. May show 'stranger shyness'. Takes stuff to mouth.	Finds feet interesting. Understand objects and know what to expect of them. Understand 'up' and 'down' and make appropriate gestures, such as raising his arms to be picked.	Double syllable sounds such as 'mama' and 'dada'. Laughs in play. Screams with annoyance.
9 Months	Sits unsupported. Grasps with thumb and index finger. Releases toys by dropping. Wiggles and crawls. Sits unsupported. Picks up objects with pincer grasp. Looks for fallen objects. Holds bottle. Is visually attentive.	Apprehensive about strangers. Imitates hand-clapping. Clings to familiar adults.	Shows interest in picture books. Watches activities of others with interest.	Babbles tunefully. Vocalises to attract attention. Enjoy communicating with sounds.
1 Year	Stands holding furniture. Stands alone for a second or two, then collapses with a bump. Walks holding one hand. Bends down and picks up objects. Pulls to stand and sits deliberately. May walk alone. Holds spoon. Points at objects. Picks up small objects.	Cooperates with dressing. Waves goodbye. Understands simple commands. Demonstrate affection. Participate in nursery rhymes.	Responds to simple instructions. Uses trial-and-error to learn about objects.	Babbles 2 or 3 words repeatedly. Responds to simple instructions. Understands several words. Uses jargon.
15 Months	Can crawl up stairs frontwards. Kneels unaided. Balance is poor. Can crawl down stairs backwards. Builds 2 block tower. Can place objects precisely. Turns pages of picture book.	Helps with dressing. Indicates soiled or wet paints. Emotionally dependent on familiar adult.	Is very curious.	Can communicate needs. Jabbers freely and loudly.
	Squats to pick up toys. Can walk alone. Drinks without spilling. Picks up toy without falling	Plays alone near familiar adult. Demands constant	Enjoys simple	Uses 'Jargon'.

PREGNANCY AND PAEDIATRICS

A CHIROPRACTIC APPROACH

ISBN 0 9551328 0 0

PREGNANCY AND PAEDIATRICS

A CHIROPRACTIC APPROACH

by
Stephen P. Williams D.C., F.C.C. (paed), F.C.C. (cranio)
Doctor of Chiropractic
Certified Craniopath

PREGNANCY AND PAEDIATRICS

A CHIROPRACTIC APPROACH

Published by
Stephen P. Williams
158 Winchester Road
Southampton
SO16 6UE

First Published 2005

Stephen P. Williams
PREGNANCY AND PAEDIATRICS: A Chiropractic Approach
Includes bibliographical, references and index

Typeset in 12pt Times New Roman

The publisher has made every effort to trace the copyright holders for borrowed material. If any has been inadvertently overlooked, the publisher will be pleased to make the necessary arrangements at the first opportunity.

Printed and Bound in Great Britain by The Print Shop, Aylesbury, Buckinghamshire HP19 9LW

Note: The Author does not assume any responsibility for any injury and/or damage to persons or property arising out of or related to any use of the material contained in this book. It is the responsibility of the treating practitioner, relying on independent experience and knowledge of the patient, to determine the best treatment and method of application for the patient.

Contents

Stephen P. Williams D.C., F.C.C. (paed), F.C.C. (cranio)

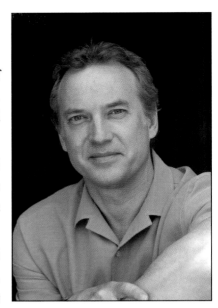

Dr Steve Williams graduated from the Anglo European College of Chiropractic (AECC) in 1987 and has practised in the UK since then. His interest in paediatrics was fuelled by the birth of his first child Tom in 1989.

He received certification in craniopathy from the International Craniopathic Society in 1996 and was made a Fellow of the College of Chiropractors (UK) Faculties of Paediatrics and Craniopathy in 2000.

Dr Williams has lectured extensively in paediatrics, sacro occipital technique and craniopathy in the United Kingdom, Australia, France, Switzerland, Germany, Greece and the USA. Along with Dr Joyce Miller, he developed the MSc in Applied Professional Development: Chiropractic Paediatrics currently running at the AECC and is heavily involved in the teaching and assessment of it. He is currently developing a postgraduate paediatric certification course with Logan Chiropractic College in the United States.

He is a past Director of Academic Affairs for the College of Chiropractors and has served on the Board of Sacro Occipital Technique Organisation Europe. Currently, he is a member of the regulatory body for chiropractic in the UK, the General Chiropractic Council.

Dr Williams runs a family-based practice in Southampton specialising in paediatrics and craniopathy.

For my family, especially my children Tom, Rachael and Megs, who showed me the way and from whom I have learnt so much.

PREGNANCY AND PAEDIATRICS A CHIROPRACTIC APPROACH

Preface

My purpose in writing this book is to provide the chiropractor with a "hands on, how to" approach to chiropractic paediatrics. When I graduated in 1987, there was very little written on the subject and my undergraduate training consisted primarily of medical paediatrics, so the learning was very much on the job. Since then, a number of chiropractic texts on paediatrics have been written that provide good sources of reference and information, but I still felt there was a need for a practical text.

While I have included some of the research regarding chiropractic care for various paediatric conditions, the focus is not on the evidence base, I will let other texts do that, instead, the focus is on my experience of the practical aspects of care with a particular focus on the function of the craniosacral system. I have quoted and used the expertise of many authorities in chiropractic, osteopathy and related fields in the text, but the interpretation is mine and my apologies to them for any changes in their original meaning.

It is my experience and strong contention that chiropractic care in its widest sense, when applied to an infant or child, will prevent or ameliorate many of the ills of childhood and later life, but that is somewhat difficult to prove in a randomised controlled trial and as such stays in the realm of opinion.

ACKNOWLEDGEMENTS

I would like to express my sincere gratitude to a number of colleagues for their encouragement with the project and help with the manuscript, they are, : Dr Simon Bird, Dr John Farmer, Dr Jonathan Howat, Dr Anthony Metcalfe and Dr Suzanne Seekins.

My appreciation also goes to Mr. John Burgess (jmbphotographic.co.uk) for the majority of the photography with additions from Dr Simon Billings. Mr. Tim Bernhard ably provided the majority of the illustrations, an unusual diversion from his normal field of natural history. My thanks also to Ms Amanda Gains for many of the skull strain illustrations.

Two individuals have contributed their significant professional expertise in the production of this book and have proved to be wonderfully helpful to the author; they are Dr Carrie Walker the proof editor and Mr. Esmond Pickering the printer at printshopuk.com.

To Miss Lesley Morgan my huge thanks for her work on typing and organising the manuscript and its author and especially for her ability to read rather challenging hand writing. Many thanks also to my colleagues and staff at St James Chiropractic Clinic for helping and putting up with me during the past year.

To those professionals who I have over the years been taught and inspired by, from both the United States and Europe my grateful thanks; there are too many to mention them all. I will however thank the individual whose example inspired me onto the path of paediatrics and craniopathy in the first place, my friend Dr Jonathan Howat. My appreciation must also go to the late Dr Major DeJarnette for the inspiration of his life's work in Sacro Occipital Technique.

Many thanks to the models for the photographs without whom the book would not have been possible (Joanna, Megan, Rachael, Lucy, Finlay, Bethany, James, Freya and Matthew).

Finally my thanks to my family for their patience and forbearance over the last 18 months, (promise I will not write another book for a while kids!)

FOREWORD

This book is in every sense a chiropractic text on paediatrics. Many authors tend to lose their way with this important subject and include a lot of irrelevant information purely because they do not understand cranial physiology.

Dr Williams has produced a manuscript which takes the Doctor of Chiropractic through the various stages of pregnancy and birth, to the examination and treatment of the neonate.

The narrative is descriptive and informative, the author using a chronological format of examination, assessment and correction in all aspects of clinical evaluation. The book has a good flow to it and is easy to understand and follow, and as is true with all well thought out text books, the illustrations and references are numerous and explicit.

The chapter on the craniosacral system is comprehensively dealt with and should encourage students to learn, understand and appreciate the physiology of this magnificent system that controls and brings about homeostasis to the central nervous system.

To attempt to be a chiropractic paediatrician without this knowledge leaves one unequipped and deficient in ones ability to evaluate and treat the paediatric patient.

Coupled with this the author dedicates a chapter to Plagiocephaly which further elaborates the necessity to be conversant with the types of fascial strains that take place in the neonatal cranium. These strains if not corrected bring about the aetiology of the dyslexic, dyspraxic and dysfunctional traits one comes across in clinical practice. One needs to understand and clarify these if one is to be successful in taking care of infants and children.

In conclusion it is my opinion that Dr Williams has used his expansive knowledge base to produce a well written and illustrated book on a vital subject, and this text should be included in every chiropractic paediatrician's library.

Jonathan Howat DC; DICS; FICS; FCC (paed) FCC (cranio)

Chapter 1
Chiropractic care during pregnancy

OVERVIEW

I regard chiropractic care during pregnancy as one of the most vital parts of paediatric chiropractic practice because it is during the time prior to birth that many of the potential traumas that can afflict the neonate may well be prevented or at least ameliorated. Birth can be the first incident in a long chain of events that gradually reduce an individual's adaptive range, and chiropractic care of the pregnant woman is able, in my experience, to prevent many injuries, although there is as yet very little hard evidence to support this.

Many women present to the chiropractic office, when pregnant, with low back pain. Although they can receive significant benefit from chiropractic care, it is preferable to begin their care prior to pregnancy. One of the major reasons for back pain in pregnancy and difficulties during labour is poor maternal musculoskeletal health. For example, if a 30-year-old woman who has a sedentary occupation and has done little exercise since school becomes pregnant, the tone and activity of her pelvic stabilising musculature (i.e. abdominals, gluteal muscles and pelvic floor) is unlikely to be in the kind of condition to tolerate the extra stresses that pregnancy entails. She may well end up suffering from significant low back pain, sciatica and abdominal and pelvic discomfort, and her child's journey into this world will also be made more difficult.

ANATOMY

Pelvic floor

The pelvic floor can be thought of as a muscular basket suspended from the pelvis. Any distortions in its bony support will change the tensions in regions of this muscular basket. The floor is pierced by three foramina: the anus, the urethra and the vagina. The floor of this muscular basket has to dilate greatly to allow delivery, and if it is twisted and distorted, owing to pelvic rotation, logic and experience indicate that the process of birth will be more difficult and traumatic for both mother and baby.

The perineum, or pelvic floor, is made up of a group of muscles and soft tissues forming the lateral and inferior walls of the pelvis (Figures 1.1 and 1.2). The lateral components are the piriformis and obturator inter-nus muscles. The inferior wall is made up of the levator ani group (the chief and strongest part being the pubococcygeus muscle, originating from the body of the pubis), coccygeus, transverse peroneal, bulbospongiosus, ischiocavernosus and anal sphincter.

As chiropractors observe every day, pelvic rotation is very common (posterior–inferior and anterior–superior, relating to the rotation of the ileum; Gonstead listing). In addition, according to Dejarnette (1984), the founder of the sacro occipital technique (SOT), a regular accompanying feature is sacroiliac instability. It has regularly been my experience to find both of these factors in pregnancy, probably because of the effects of pregnancy hormones on the ligamentous system and excessive and incorrect sitting postures, which are so much a part of our modern lifestyle. It seems likely that, if such posterior–inferior and anterior–superior pelvic rotation is present, particularly if it is accompanied by sacroiliac ligamentous laxity or instability, a buckling or torsion of the pelvic floor will follow, creating a more difficult passage to be traversed during birth process.

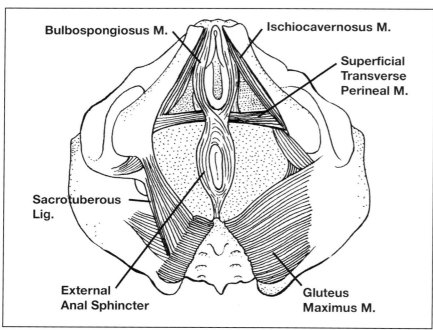

Figure 1.1 Female perineum – superficial muscles adapted from Barral and Roth: Urogenital Manipulation.

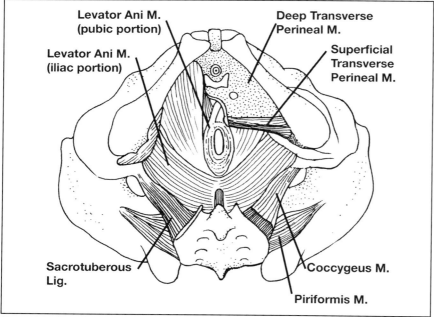

Figure 1.2   Female perineum – deep muscles adapted from Barral and Roth: Urogenital Manipulation.

Pelvic and uterine ligaments

The connection and attachment of the pelvic organs is simpler than that of the abdominal organs: there is no mesentery or double serous membrane, connection instead being made by ligaments. These ligaments contain contractile fibres, the degree of contractility being affected by general body tonus and hormone levels, especially those of progesterone.

The *uterosacral ligament* originates from the anterior sacrum, encompasses the rectum and inserts into the lower third of the uterus (Figure 1.3). The *transverse cervical ligament* has a broad origin from the ilia and inserts into the lower uterus and cervix. The *pubovesicular ligament* connects the pubis to the bladder (Figure 1.4).

As can be seen from Figure 1.5, the supporting mechanism for the cervix and upper vagina is formed by a tendinous arch of pelvic fascia bilaterally where the pelvic organs penetrate the pelvic floor. It is this support system that may well play a key role in creating a torque upon the cervix and lower uterine segment in response to distortions of the pelvic ring. Figure 1.5 above clearly shows the strong attachment of these pelvic ligaments to the sacrum, ilia and pubic bones, and it takes little imagination to envisage the consequences of pelvic distortions to these support structures and the uterus itself.

A ligament of great importance during pregnancy is the *round ligament* (Figure 1.6), which arises from the upper, outer edge of the uterus just anterior to the fallopian tube, and passes laterally within the broad ligament, through the inguinal ring and into the labium majus. It can play a role in groin pain in pregnancy and may well be involved in any torque stresses to which the uterus is exposed. It is not easily palpable except in the inguinal canal until around the

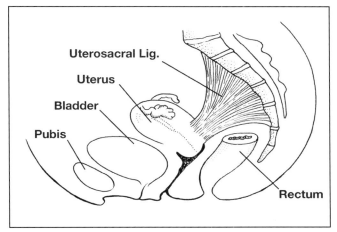

Figure 1.3 Uterosacral ligament.

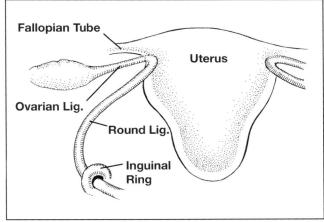

Figure 1.6 Round ligament.

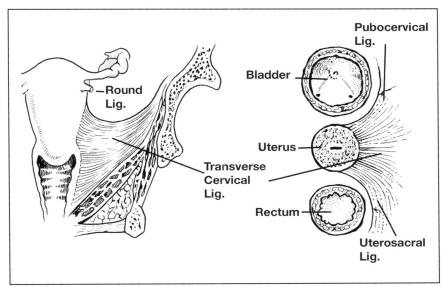

Figure 1.4 Transverse cervical ligament.

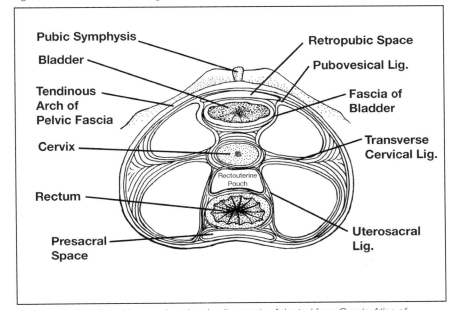

Figure 1.5 Female pelvis – section showing ligaments. Adapted from Grants Atlas of Anatomy. Kelly P.J ed

fifth month of gestation, when the uterus enlarges from the pelvis into the abdominal cavity.

FETAL POSITIONING

The fetus, as it develops towards term, is bounded above by the thoracic diaphragm and below by the pelvic diaphragm. Distortions of either of these transverse fascial planes will logically limit the ability of the fetus to move within its environment and subsequently affect its lie and freedom of movement, particularly during the last trimester.

Sutton and Scott (1996), in their excellent text, emphasised the importance of maternal posture during the last weeks of pregnancy to encourage the fetus to take up an occiput anterior position at the start of labour. They believe that the lowered level of physical activity as a result of our modern lifestyle is a major negative influence on fetal position. In particular, sitting in a modern armchair or sofa tips the pelvis backwards, a situation that is further aggravated by the woman crossing her legs and significantly decreases the space available for the fetus in the anterior part of the pelvis. Sutton and Scott regard this limitation of space as a major cause of an occiput posterior presentation, which is a common precursor of dystocia and instrumental delivery (Fan et al 1997, Fitzpatrick et al 2001). Postures and exercises to avoid this occurring are detailed in Figure 1.7.

It is also recommended (Sutton and Scott 1996) that, when nearing full term and preferably for the last trimester, women avoid:

- relaxing in a semirecumbent position with their knees higher than their hips, which causes the angle of the lumbar spine to the pelvic brim to be reduced to around 90 degrees. If a woman uses these postures regularly at the stage when the fetus is entering the pelvic brim, it is likely that – if it enters at all – it will be in the posterior part of the pelvis and therefore more likely to present as an occiput posterior;

- avoiding long car trips as modern bucket-type seats have the same effect as modern furniture;

- sitting with their legs crossed as this reduces the space available for the fetus in the anterior part of the pelvis;

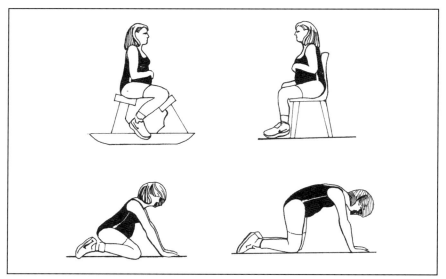

Figure 1.7 Positions and exercises for pregnancy. Adapted from Sutton and Scott: Optimum Foetal Positioning.

- squatting, which is not advisable in late pregnancy unless the fetus has engaged in the pelvic brim. Deep squatting can encourage an occiput posterior fetus to engage before it has had a chance to change to occiput anterior.

INTRAUTERINE CONSTRAINT

After the seventh month of gestation, any position other than vertex in an attitude of flexion is considered to create some degree of constraint (Forrester and Anrig 1998).

I will look at the causes of constraint with an emphasis on the biomechanical causes, which we as chiropractors hope to influence.

Pelvic contracture

Pelvic contracture can create dystocia during labour; there may be contractions of the pelvic inlet, the mid-pelvis, the pelvic outlet or any combination of these. The pelvic inlet is considered to be contracted if the shortest anteroposterior diameter is less than 10 cm or the greatest transverse diameter is less than 12 cm. The contracted mid-pelvis is more common than the contracted inlet. This is present when the interischial spinous diameter is less than 8 cm. A contracted pelvic outlet is present when the interischial tuberous diameter is less than 8 cm (Cunningham et al 2001).

Distortions of the bony pelvis, although common in the early years of the 20th century owing to the prevalence of rickets, with up to 15% of women presenting at the John Hopkins Hospital, USA, in 1924 showing distortions caused by rickets (Cunningham et al 2001), are less common now. The American College of Obstetricians and Gynaecologists (1995) suggests that the bony pelvis is not, with rare exceptions, the only factor that limits vaginal delivery.

Soft tissue constraint

Uterine malformations can cause intrauterine constraint. These include varying degrees of unicornuate or bicornuate uterus and uterine septal defects (Cunningham et al 2001). Fetal wastage may be up to 40%, and the smaller uterine size is almost certainly an explanation for the increased rates of preterm delivery, fetal growth restrictions, breech presentation, dysfunctional labour and increased caesarean deliveries (Fedele et al 1987, Andrews and Jones 1998). Fetal deformations including limb deficiency, polydactyly, plagiocephaly and body wall defects have been associated with structural uterine abnormalities (Miller et al 1979, Miller 1983).

Uterine tumours such as leiomyomas have been associated with an increased incidence of fetal malpresentation, particularly when they involve the lower uterine segment. Because of the difficulties of performing an external version or vaginal delivery, they are considered to be an indicator for caesarean section (Bruk and Sherer 1997).

The literature is somewhat equivocal about the importance of placental location. In a study of 228 breech presentations published

in 1984, Luterkort et al found no evidence of cornufundal placental location. However, in a more recent study by Filipov et al (2000) of 124 breech presentations, 62.6% showed a cornufundal placental location, whereas this was present in only 4.8% of the vertex-presenting group. An anterior placental location has been linked to occiput posterior presentations at term (Gardberg and Tuppurainen 1994).

Maternal abdominal tone is also a factor. Laxity of the maternal abdominal wall from high parity has an association with a higher rate of fetal malpresentation. Women who have had four or more deliveries have a 10-fold increase in the incidence of a transverse lie compared with nulliparous women (Cunningham et al 2001). The mechanism appears to be a relaxation of the abdominal wall with a pendulous abdomen that allows the uterus to fall forwards, deflecting the long axis of the fetus away from the axis of the birth canal.

It is interesting to speculate whether the decreased abdominal tone that is found in generally sedentary workers may have a detrimental effect on fetal position in a wider number of pregnancies and whether this may be one of the factors for the much greater number of interventions performed in current obstetric practice.

The fetus

Fetal factors involved in intrauterine constraint include excessive fetal size, multiple pregnancy, hydrocephaly and anencephaly (Anrig and Plaugher 1998). Oligohydramnios and polyhydramnios are also associated with an increase in malpresentation (Luterkort et al 1984).

It has also been suggested that strong fetal movements are necessary for the fetus to position itself properly (Suzuki and Yamamuro 1985). The investigators postulated that fetal version occurs as the fetus attempts to accommodate itself to the shape of the uterus during the active state of whole-body movements, and that malpresentation will occur if these movement are weak or absent.

Unknown aetiology

Luterkort et al (1984) noted that although there was a reason for some of the fetal constraint they observed, 85% was of unknown aetiology. It seems probable that at least some of this figure may originate from biomechanical constraint. If the ilia rotate, they can cause tension through the transverse cervical ligaments. If the sacrum, as commonly happens, subluxates in an anterior–inferior direction, this will stress the uterosacral ligament, creating stress on the lower third of the uterus and the cervix. This will surely have the potential to affect the freedom of movement of the fetus. If this is further compounded by twisting of the pelvic floor and respiratory diaphragm – the two transverse fascial planes either side of the near-term fetus – we should not be surprised if constraint is the result.

Unfortunately, we have only theory to support the conjecture that biomechanical constraint could have its origin in pelvic and sacral subluxations causing stress on the uterus and transverse fascial planes (diaphragms) above and below. There is, however, at least some evidence, even though it does not totally stand up to critical appraisal, that chiropractic care is effective in the treatment of intrauterine constraint.

In a survey of chiropractors, Pistolese (2002) showed a 92% success rate in correcting breech presentations using the Webster breech technique. It would seem likely however that those chiropractors who have had successful outcomes with their care would be more willing to reply to the survey In addition, Kanau (1998) published a study of six case reports, all of late breech presentation converted to vertex presentation using the same technique. Fetal position however was only identified using the Leopold manoeuvres and not by ultrasonic examination. There

are many more reports, both in the literature and anecdotally, of chiropractic care correcting fetal malposition. In the author's own experience of some 20 cases in recent years, the success rate approaches 90%.

Case report

A 30-year-old nulliparous female presented with a 37-week gestation pregnancy in a transverse lie, identified on ultrasonic examination. The fetus had been in this lie throughout the third trimester. The woman was due to be admitted to hospital the following day as a precaution against spontaneous labour and was due for a caesarean section in 10 days' time.

On examination, vital signs were normal, and neurological and orthopaedic examinations were within normal limits. Palpatory examination revealed the fetal head in the right upper quadrant under the maternal liver and the lower limbs in the lower left quadrant.

Chiropractic examination revealed a sacroiliac instability on the right, with a right anterior inferior sacrum. The right side of the diaphragm was hypertonic and immobile, as was the left pelvic floor. The round ligament on the left was hypertonic and prominent to palpation.

Clinical impression. Intrauterine constraint was causing an oblique fetal presentation owing to pelvic instability, sacral

torsion and accompanying hypertonicity of sections of the superior and inferior transverse fascial planes.

Treatment. The sacrum was adjusted prone (with the woman on a pregnancy pillow), and soft tissue releases were performed to the right psoas, the respiratory diaphragm and the pelvic floor. The patient was then blocked supine (SOT category II).

Outcome. The patient reported by phone the next day that ultrasound examination revealed that the fetus was now in a vertex presentation. The planned hospitalisation was cancelled, and the patient received two more chiropractic adjustments prior to labour. At 39.5 weeks, a healthy 3.63 kg (8 lb) baby was delivered on the lounge floor at home – the labour had been so fast that the paramedics had no time to get the woman to hospital.

LEOPOLD MANOEUVRES

In 1894, Leopold and Sporlin described a systematic palpatory examination of the pregnant abdomen using four manoeuvres that is still in widespread use today (Cunningham et al 2001). According to Lydon-Rochelle et al (1993), experienced clinicians can accurately identify fetal malpresentation using the Leopold manoeuvres with a high sensitivity (88%), specificity (94%), positive predictive value (74%)

and negative predictive value (97%). The clinicians involved in this research were midwives; chiropractors, with their years of training in palpatory skills, should not find learning and using these manoeuvres beyond them, and indeed they are an essential skill for the chiropractor wishing to treat pregnant mothers.

The mother lies supine with her abdomen exposed. During the first three manoeuvres, the examiner faces the patient's head; during the fourth manoeuvre, it is easier to face the woman's feet (Figure 1.8d). It should be remembered that if the patient is very obese or has an anteriorly located placenta, palpation maybe very difficult or impossible.

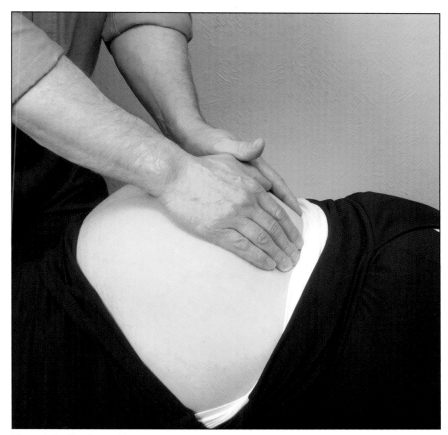

Figure 1.8a First Leopold manoeuvre.

First manoeuvre

After outlining the contour of the uterus and assessing how close the uterine fundus is to the xiphoid cartilage, the examiner gently palpates the fundus using the tips of both hands (Figure 1.8a). The examiner tries to differentiate which fetal pole is present in the fundus. The breech gives the sensation of a large round nodular body, whereas the head feels hard and round, and is more easily moveable and ballotable.

Second manoeuvre

After determining which pole is present in the fundus, the palms are placed on either side of the abdomen, and a gentle but

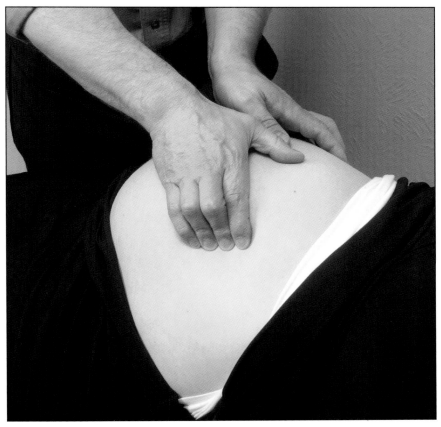

Figure 1.8b Second Leopold manoeuvre.

deep pressure is exerted (Figure 1.8b). The tips of the fingers can be brought into play for greater sensitivity. The examiner is trying to differentiate between, on one side, a hard resistant structure – the fetal back and spine – and on the other, several small mobile parts, which are the fetal extremities. In the presence of obesity or excess amniotic fluid, this may be difficult and require counter pressure to identify the fetal back. Some indication of the orientation of the fetus can be made from noting whether the back is directed to the anterior, posterior or lateral aspect, or transversely.

Third manoeuvre

Using the thumb and forefingers nearest the patient, the examiner grasps the maternal abdomen just above the pubic symphysis (Figure 1.8c); if the presenting part is not engaged, a movable body (hopefully the head) will be felt. Differentiation between the head and the breech is made as in the first manoeuvre. If the presenting part is deeply engaged, the findings simply indicate that the lower fetal pole is fixed in the pelvis. If the fetal head can be identified, careful palpation can demonstrate the attitude of the head. If the cephalic prominence is on the same side as the extremities, the head is flexed; if it is on the same side as the fetal back; the head is extended. This is confirmed by the fourth manoeuvre.

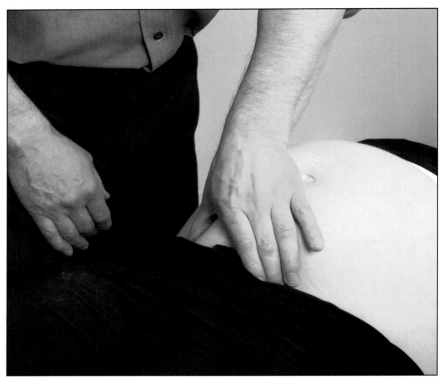

Figure 1.8c Third Leopold manoeuvre.

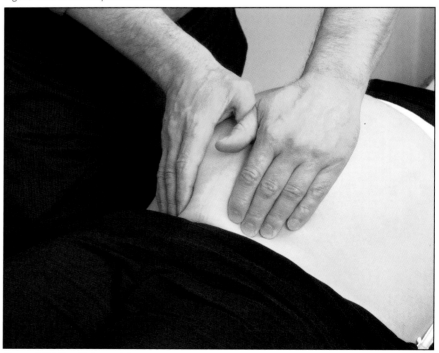

Figure 1.8d Fourth Leopold manoeuvre.

Fourth manoeuvre

The examiner faces the mother's feet and, with the fingertips of both hands, exerts a gentle but deep pressure towards the pelvic inlet (Figure 1.8d). If the head is the presenting part, one of the examiner's hands is arrested before than the other by a rounded body – the cephalic prominence – whereas the other hand descends more deeply into the pelvis. If the presentation is vertex (neck flexion), the prominence is on the same side as the extremities. In a face or brow presentation, the prominence is on the same side as the fetal back.

CHIROPRACTIC CARE IN PREGNANCY

As mentioned above, chiropractic care is best begun in preparation for pregnancy. If the sacrum, pelvis and transverse fascial planes are balanced prior to the woman becoming pregnant, the management will logically be easier and the chance of constraint will be lessened. Advance planning is not, however, commonly the case, and many women seek care only because of symptoms of musculoskeletal pain or because malpositions become evident in the third trimester. Prior to or in the first two trimesters of pregnancy, care should be directed towards maintaining the balance and stability of the pelvic ring (sacroiliac joints and pubic symphysis) and balancing the tone of the diaphragm and pelvic floor. This should not be the only area undergoing care: a whole-body approach is important. As chiropractors, we should be only too well aware that distortions in any one transverse fascial plane are capable of causing compensatory distortions in other transverse facial planes.

There is some evidence of the efficacy of chiropractic care decreasing the mean duration of labour. Fallon (1991), in a comparative study of 65 women undergoing chiropractic care through pregnancy, showed a 24% shorter labour time in primagravidae and 39% shorter labour times in muligravid subjects.

Transverse fascial plane release

The transverse fascial planes are those planes of tissue running horizontally across the body when we look at a standing subject. They include the cranial dural membranes, the thoracic outlet, the respiratory diaphragm and the pelvic floor. When considering pregnancy, the last two are the most important.

Psoas assessment and release should be undertaken first as the iliopsoas group originates in part from the crura of the diaphragm and restriction will affect diaphragmatic function.

Stretch the supine patient's arms overhead as far as possible in line with his or her nose and look for arm shortening (Figure 1.9). This can indicate a restricted psoas muscle on that side. Release the psoas by standing at the side of

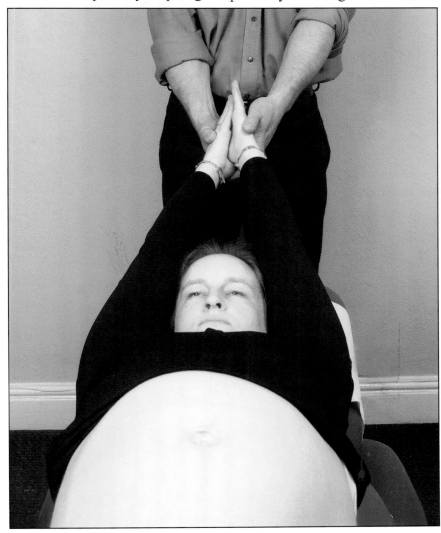

Figure 1.9 Psoas evaluation showing a right psoas contracture.

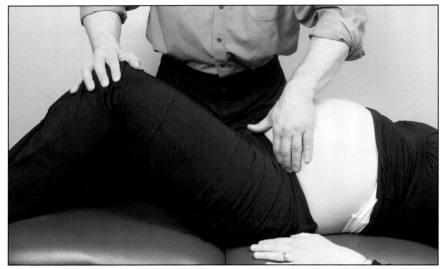

Figure 1.10 Left psoas release.

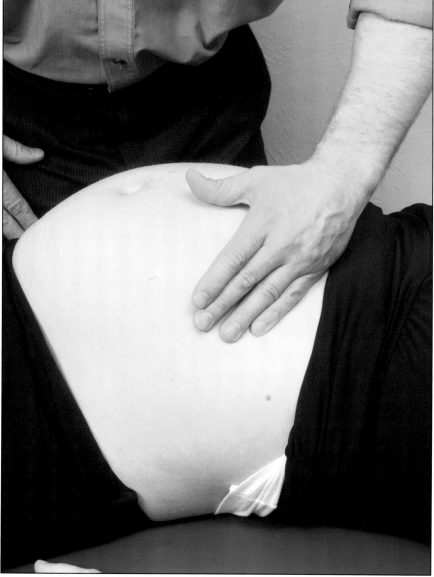

Figure 1.11 Diaphragm assessment.

the patient opposite the side of restriction and flex the leg of the involved side with the foot flat on the bench. Stabilise that leg with the lower hand, and with your upper hand come in medially to the opposite anterior superior iliac spine lateral to the fetus and stretch the tissues in a superior to inferior and inferior to superior direction (Figure 1.10).

This should result in an evening-out of the arms' lengths, but you may find that you now have to release the other side. If after this there is a persistent arm length discrepancy, this can mean the diaphragm is hypertonic on that side or that there is a kidney ptosis present on that side.

Diaphragm release

The SOT indicator for a hypertonic diaphragm is nodulation in the ipsilateral sternocleidomastoid at the level of cervical vertebrae C4–C5. The soft tissues just under the anterior border of the ribs are palpated for hypertonicity, indicating diaphragmatic tightness (Figure 1.11).

The release is performed with the thumbs opposed at their tips. Tissue entry is initially gained under the ribs by following them in deep inspiration as they rise and holding that position as they fall in expiration. This initial 'slow stretch' gains tissue entry, and once that has been accomplished the thumbs are pulled apart and away in a splint or 'fast-stretch' technique (Figure 1.12). This may need to be performed in several areas to gain diaphragm relaxation. The nodulation of the sternocleidomastoid should be greatly reduced.

Hiatus hernia technique

Many women get symptoms of gastric or oesophageal reflux during pregnancy. This can be simply due to the mechanical stresses and pressure encountered by the diaphragm and the oesophagus. For many women, correction can be attained by decreasing the tension and stress on the cardiac portion of the stomach. The SOT indicator is nodulation on the left anterior third rib in the mid-nipple line.

For correction, the patient lies supine with the knees comfortably bent and the feet flat on the bench. The doctor stands on the right-hand side of the bench. The contact is made with reinforced fingers under the anterior ribs near the xiphoid process, pointing to the patient's left shoulder. On full inspiration, the fingers follow under the ribs towards the left shoulder, and on expiration a clockwise torque (towards the left iliac fossa) is introduced. This slow stretch is repeated several times, gathering more and more tissue in a clockwise torque (slow stretch) and not allowing the tension gathered to release. The release comes at the beginning of an inspiration with a small fast-stretch torque further in the

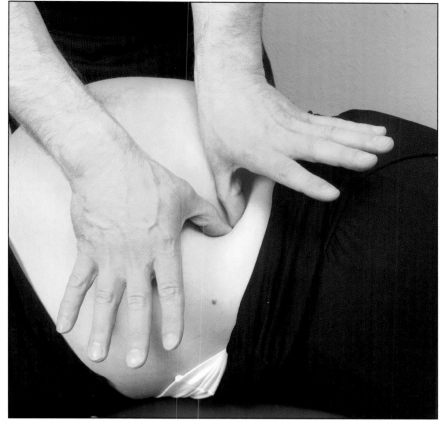

Figure 1.12a Diaphragm release.

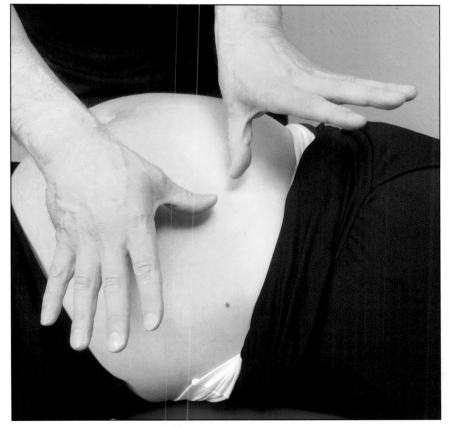

Figure 1.12b Diaphragm release finish.

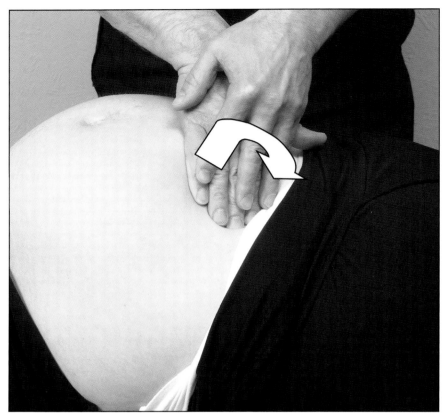

Figure 1.13a Hiatus hernia correction, arrow showing direction of tissue manipulation.

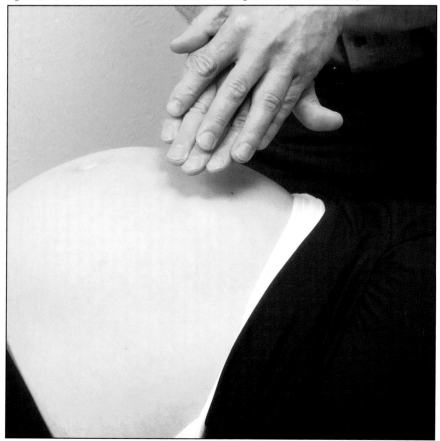

Figure 1.13.b Hiatus hernia correction, post release.

clockwise direction (Figure 1.13). The nodulation on the left third rib should be reduced.

It should be remembered that this technique needs to be performed gently and specifically so as not to stress the fetus. It is easier to perform early in pregnancy rather than at the end of the last trimester.

Kidney lift

Kidney ptosis is a common clinical finding in pregnancy and often follows chronic psoas hypertonicity as these two structures are enveloped in the same fascial bundle. This correction also seems to allow the kidneys to increase their fluid drainage and can be useful in some cases of fluid retention.

The indicator is a short arm on the overhead psoas test that is resistive to correction. Correction is made with the woman lying on her side, involved side upwards, which is helpful as it moves the fetus out of the way. The patient flexes both legs to 90 degrees. The doctor stands behind the patient and contacts the tissues medial to the anterior superior iliac spine under the kidney with the other hand supporting posteriorly just above the iliac crest (Figure 1.14a). The woman is instructed to inhale deeply, which results in the diaphragm pushing the abdominal soft tissue inferiorly, and then exhale fully. This causes the abdominal soft tissues including the kidneys to rebound and follow the diaphragm as it moves superiorly. The doctor's hands emphasise this movement and hold the soft tissues inferior to the kidney in a superior direction. This may take two repetitions.

The doctor then instructs the patient to straighten her legs on exhalation while he or she holds the soft tissues in a cephalic or superior direction (Figure 1.14b). This may be further emphasised by getting the patient to move her ipsilateral arm above her head (Figure 1.14c). The lift is then completed, but it may need correction on the other side as well as this is often now the short arm on the overhead test.

Pelvic floor balancing

Pelvic floor balancing is a very gentle technique that uses an indirect fascial release adjustment rather than direct stretches because of the proximity of the fetus and the possibility of injury with forceful adjustments in this area.

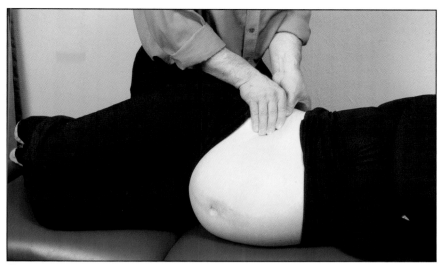

Figure 1.14a Kidney lift, gentle cephalic traction is applied.

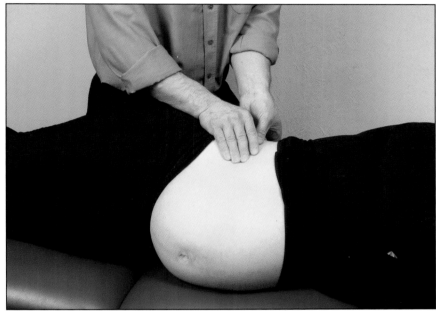

Figure 1.14b Kidney lift, the patient straightens her legs, the doctor holds the cephalic traction.

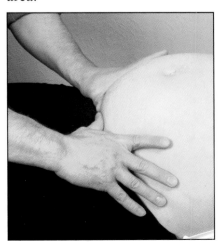

Figure 1.15 Pelvic floor balancing.

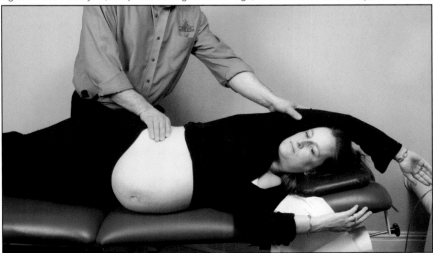

Figure 1.14c Kidney lift, the doctor holds cephalic traction with one hand and stretches the patients arm away from the inferior contact.

13

The patient lies supine with her knees comfortably bent. The doctor contacts the soft tissues at the superior aspect of the pubis with the thumb tips opposed in the centre of the pubic symphysis (Figure 1.15). The thumbs are spread out along the top of the pubic bones, contacting as much tissue as possible. Very gently, lift these tissues in a cephalic direction with a few ounces of pressure, assessing the resistance of the tissues. Any area of tightness or restriction is released in the direction of its easiest motion; this may be superior, inferior, medial, lateral, with a twist or oblique. The tissue is followed rather than led into correction. The process is an unwinding and may take a minute or so. The adjustment is complete when tissue pliability is gained in all directions, particularly lifting cephalically.

This type of adjustment may be new to many chiropractors as it involves an indirect rather than a direct approach, but it is worth mastering as the therapeutic effects are, in my experience, marked.

The piriformis muscles

It is of great importance that these muscles are kept in reasonable condition during pregnancy because of their insertion on to the sacrum. Any hypertonicity will tend to create a posterior rotational stress on the sacrum on the same side. They are also the most common cause of sciatica in pregnancy, true disc lesions being rare because of the effect of the pregnancy hormones on the intervertebral discs. Bilateral piriformis contracture causes a band-like pain at the level of the sacrum and buttocks in pregnancy.

It is a good idea to teach the pregnant woman's partner to give a regular side-lying massage to the buttock muscles in general and the piriformis group in particular. In the clinic, releases can consist of any technique that the chiropractor is comfortable with as long as the result is to keep the muscles balanced and relaxed.

Sacral assessment and correction

There are many methods of assessing and correcting the sacrum, the primary issue

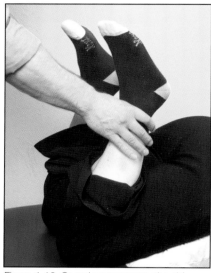

Figure 1.16 Sacral assessment, the side reduced knee flexion is the side of sacral posteriority.

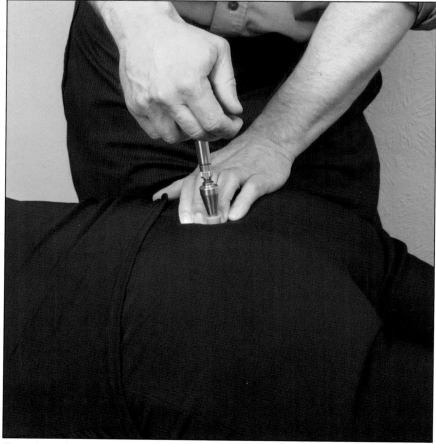

Figure 1.17a Sacral correction: posterior side , with an activator.

being that any anterior or posterior torsion of the sacrum is diagnosed and adjusted. The following method is therefore not the only one, but it is a useful and low-force method.

The patient lies prone; after 4–5 months' gestation it is necessary to use either an adjusting table with a 'breakaway' abdominal section or a pregnancy pillow. The sacrum is assessed by flexing both heels to the buttocks and checking which side is more resistant, leading to a greater heel-to-buttock distance (Figure 1.16). This is commonly the side of the posterior sacrum.

The adjustment is via an activator on all five sacral segments on

the side of posteriority (Figure 1.17a). This is followed by a flat-hand contact on the sacrum, using a vibratory pressure through the line of the sacroiliac joint on

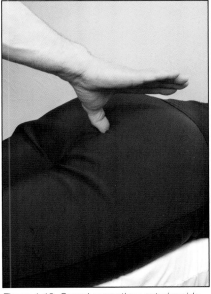

Figure 1.18 Sacral correction: anterior side - Logan basic, sacrotuberous ligament contact.

the side of the posterior sacrum (Figure 1.17b). If this does not totally correct the sacrum, a Logan basic adjustment is given on the anterior sacral side (Figure 1.18).

Pubic symphysis

The pubic symphysis is an often forgotten but very important part of the three-joint complex that forms the pelvic ring and is an area that often becomes unstable during pregnancy. Symphysis pubis dysfunction is a common cause of pain and disability in pregnancy and very much within the remit of the chiropractor to treat effectively.

The easiest method of checking the function and stability of the pubic symphysis is to test the strength of the adductor muscles in three positions: toes together with heels out, heels together with toes out and conventionally with the feet together (Figure 1.19). This variation changes

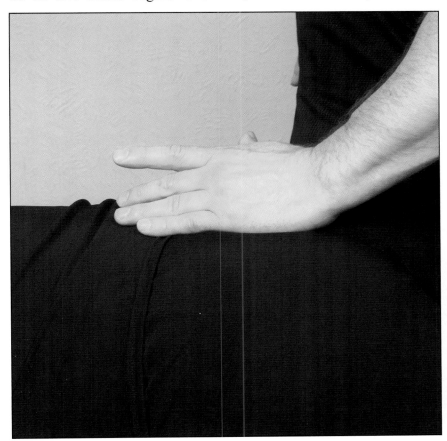

Figure 1.17b Sacral correction: posterior side.

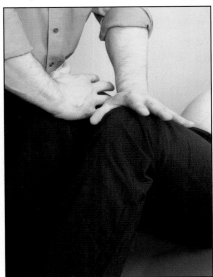

Figure 1.19 Pubic symphysis: adductor test.

the vectors of force travelling through the symphysis via the adductor muscles, and alignment or stability problems either show up as muscle weakness and/or pain on one or more of the tests.

If there is a subluxation at the symphysis in pregnancy, it will tend to be very tender so the technique of choice that often works is the use of resisted knee abduction/adduction. The woman should be instructed to push with about a third of her strength, the doctor first resisting the movement and then letting go suddenly (Figure 1.20). This often allows the pubic symphysis to reset, and it is worth trying two or three of these resisted movements before retesting the previously discovered weakness.

In my experience, more than 80% of cases will correct; if they do not, the use of an activator may be effective. The best method appears to be contacting the side of the high pubis with the thumb and activating the pubis via the thumb (Figure 1.21a). The direction of application is caudal, and it is recommended that the pubis be divided into three sections, each being treated separately to gain the best result. The inferior ramus should be adjusted in the same way in a cephalic direction (Figure 1.21b). Be aware that even this seemingly gentle adjustment can be uncomfortable for the patient with a disrupted pubic symphysis.

Another option is a technique in which the patient's knee and

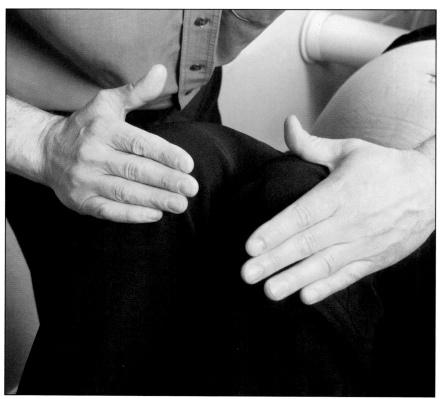

Figure 1.20 Indirect method of pubic symphysis correction.

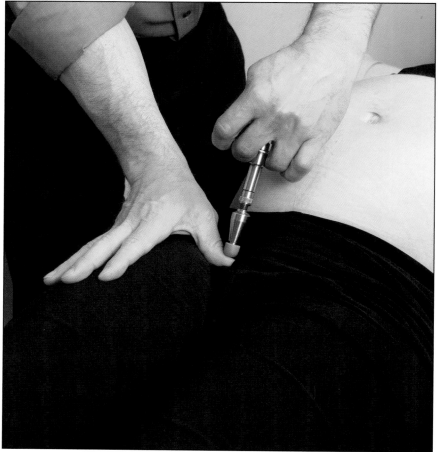

Figure 1.21a Pubic symphysis. Activation of the superior ramus.

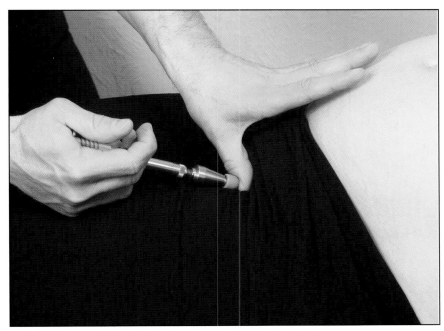

Figure 1.21b Pubic symphysis. Activation of the inferior ramus.

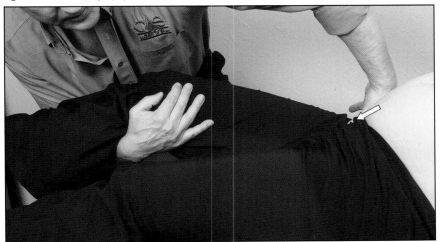

Figure 1.22a Pubic symphysis. Manual correction of the superior ramus.

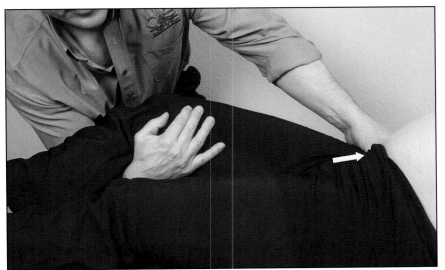

Figure 1.22b Pubic symphysis. Manual correction of the inferior ramus.

hip are flexed to 90 degrees and a thumb contact is taken on the ramus to be corrected. As the leg is slowly straightened by the doctor, the ramus is gently but firmly pressed into the direction of correction, which can be superior to inferior or inferior to superior depending on the direction of subluxation (Figure 1.22).

Pelvic instability

This topic is covered in depth by SOT seminars, so it will be touched on only briefly here. Any instability affecting the sacroiliac joints will often allow the sacrum to twist – earlier in the chapter, we looked at the significant effect that this might have on the soft tissues of the pelvis and therefore the fetus.

One of the simplest tests to perform to find out whether instability is present is the standing stress test devised by Hochman (1999). The standing patient puts both her arms straight out in front, and the doctor tests the strength in a floor-wards direction. The patient's weight is then orientated on to first one foot and then the other, testing again; any weakening indicates an unstable sacroiliac joint on that side (Figure 1.23). For those experienced in SOT, this can supplement the arm fossa test; for those who are not SOT practitioners, it will give a strong indication of pelvic instability.

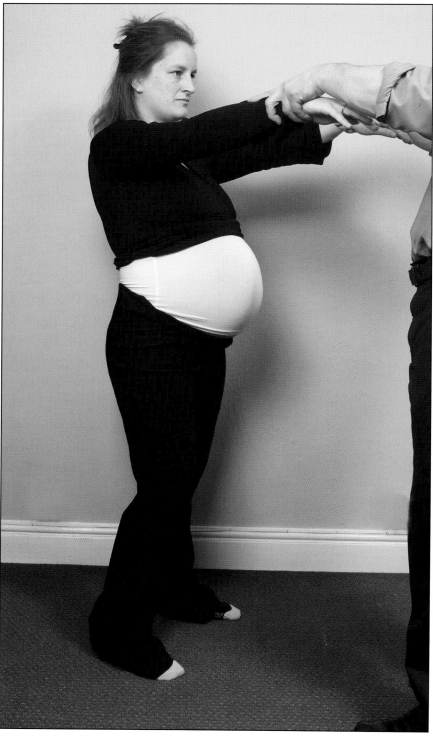

Figure 1.23 Standing stress test.

Premature labour

It can be a very difficult task to identify any specific causative factor for premature labour. Phillips (2001) has developed a theory that posterior subluxations of individual sacral segments may put tension on the uterosacral ligament and therefore traction on the cervix, causing prostaglandin release that starts early labour. Although this is purely theoretical, it has been my experience that correcting the posterior sacral segments can halt the contractions of premature labour. This subluxation pattern in the sacrum appears to be mainly post-traumatic in origin.

To assess this, the woman is asked to stand facing a wall about 60 cm (2 feet) from it, legs apart and with her hands against the wall as if she is about to be frisked! The doctor stands by her side with one hand supporting under the pregnant abdomen. The other hand, fingers pointing to the floor, slides down on the heel of the hand from the lumbar spine on to the sacrum (Figure 1.24a). Any sacral posteriority tends to arrest the hand's progress. This is then released using a fascial release technique (Figure 1.24b).

The hand contacting the sacrum tries to find the free direction of movement of the restriction, whether it be superior, medial, lateral, a twist or in an oblique direction. This is then followed in the direction of free movement

The easiest and least stressful way (for the patient) to correct this is to use supine blocks. The short leg is treated with the block under the iliac crest at a right angle to it, and the long leg is blocked under the greater trochanter at an angle of 45 degrees. The blocking should take no more than a couple of minutes.

until a release is obtained; the hand will then slide freely down the sacrum.

Due to the pregnancy and subsequent hormone levels, this will need repeating, and it is often worth teaching the woman's partner how to do this manoeuvre as it may need daily correction.

Although I do not believe that this will help every case of premature labour, it is worth trying as success means an avoidance of a lengthy hospital stay, the possibility of premature delivery and the damage that this might entail to the fetus.

Labour

It is always worth talking to the patient and her partner about the labour and strategies that they might use to allow it to proceed in the easiest and least traumatic way with the lowest possibility of intervention. It is important both to educate and to empower them as birth in the hospital setting can be a very intimidating event. They should be encouraged to have a birth plan in which they can actively assist labour to progress rather than wait for events to overtake them.

Gravity is one of the best means of assistance in early labour so walking, standing or leaning on the partner should be encouraged. The patient should be advised to avoid lying (except side-lying), semireclining positions and sitting (Sutton and Scott 1996) as these positions decrease the

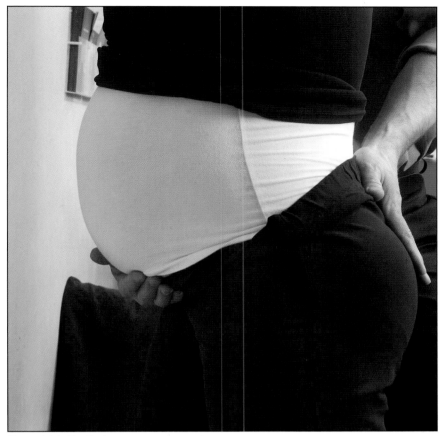

Figure 1.24a Buckled sacrum: assessment.

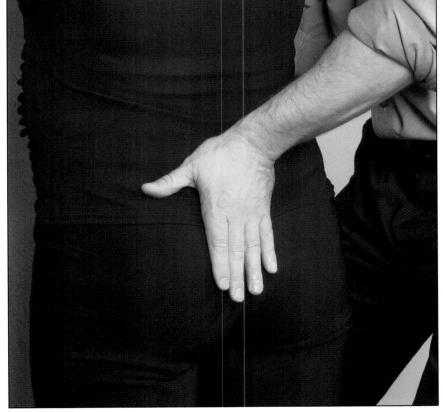

Figure 1.24b Buckled sacrum: correction.

anteroposterior pelvic diameter and can mean that the fetus has to pass 'uphill'.

If the fetus' head is stuck in an asynclistic position, the woman should be encouraged to put one foot up on a small stool or the stairs and gently rock the pelvis from side to side (Sutton and Scott 1996).

A maternal anterior sacral base can be a problem by preventing descent and internal rotation. When this occurs, the mother will very often feel the pain during contractions, particularly in her low back. A useful technique to teach the partner is a sacral apex stretch (Figure 1.25). This is performed with the woman on all fours, the partner pushing with the heel of their hand on the sacral apex. This position should be held for several minutes (at least two contractions), or longer if it is helpful, and the woman should then be encouraged to get up and walk about.

Phillips (2001) recommends a side-lying technique to reduce back-labour (Figure 1.26). The woman lies on her side at the edge of the bed with her head on a pillow, and her partner stands facing the bed to support her. It is important that the woman's spine is kept straight and level, her top leg being stabilised between her partner's legs and allowed to gently fall towards the floor. Her partner holds her shoulder and hip so that she cannot fall. This position is held for several minutes and then repeated on

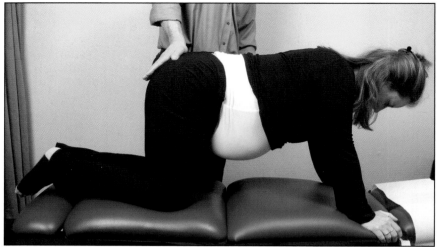

Figure 1.25 Dystocia treatment – sacral apex stretch.

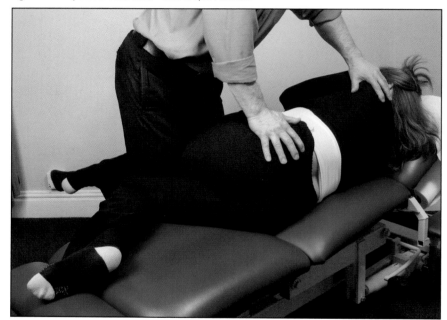

Figure 1.26 Dystocia treatment – side-lying pelvic stretch.

the other side. The woman will be generally aware if this has helped her, and labour should proceed more easily.

If the side-lying technique does not help, the technique used for the anterior sacral base can again be used but this time with the woman's pelvis raised higher, her knees resting on three pillows and her forearms flat on the bed with her head resting on them. This has the effect of changing the fluid dynamics around the

baby and the umbilical cord. Phillips (2001) recommends that, with a home delivery, this be done using the bottom of the staircase.

It is very important to empower a woman and her partner with a birth plan, so that when they are in hospital (where most deliveries still take place) they feel that they are taking an active part in the process and not just letting it happen to them.

References

American College of Obstetrics and Gynaecologists. Dystocia and the Augmentation of Labour. *Technical Bulletin No 218*. Washington: ACOG, 1995.

Andrews MC, Jones HW Jr. Impaired reproductive performance of unicornate uterus: intrauterine growth retardation, infertility and recurrent abortion. *Am J Obstet Gynecol* 1998; 91: 939.

Anrig CA, Plaugher G (eds). *Pediatric Chiropractic*. Baltimore: Williams & Wilkins, 1998.

Barral J.P. and Roth J. *Urogenital Manipulation*. Seattle: Eastland Press, 1993.

Bruk LR, Sherer DM. Intrapartum sonography of the lower uterine segments in patients with breech presenting fetuses. *Am J Perinatol* 1997; 14: 315.

Cunningham GF, Gant NF, Leveno KJ, Gilstrap LC, Hauth JC, Wenstrom KD. *Williams' Obstetrics, 21st edn*. New York: McGraw-Hill, 2001.

DeJarnette MB. *Sacro Occipital Technique*. Private publication, Nebraska, 1984.

Fallon J. The effect of chiropractic treatment on pregnancy and labour: a comprehensive study. *Proceedings of the World Chiropractic Congress*, 1991; 24–31.

Fan L, Huang X, Wang Q. The characteristics of labour course and perinatal prognosis in cases of fetal persistent occiput – transverse and persistent occiput – posterior position. *Zhonghua Fu Chan Ke Za Zhi* 1997; 32: 620–622.

Fedele L, Zamberletti D, Vermicellini P, Dota M, Candiana GB. Reproductive performance of women with unicornate uterus. *Fertil Steril* 1987; 47: 416.

Filipov E, Borisov I, Kolarov G. Placental location and its influences on the position of the fetus in the uterus: *Akush Ginekol* (Sofia) 2000; 40: 11.

Fitzpatrick M., McQuillan K, Oherlity C. Influence of persistent occiput posterior position on delivery outcome. *Obstet Gynecol* 2001; 98: 1027–1031.

Forrester JA, Anrig CA. The prenatal and perinatal period. In *Paediatric Chiropractic*, Anrig CA, Plagher G (eds). Baltimore: Williams & Wilkins, 1998.

Gardberg M, Tuppurainen M. Anterior placental location predisposes for occiput posterior presentation near term. *Acta Obstet Gynaecol Scand* 1994; 73: 51.

Hochman J. *Sacro Occipital Technique Seminar*, Omaha, Nebraska, 1999.

Kanau PL. Application of the Webster inutero constraint technique: AK series. *J Clin Chiropr Pediatr* 1998; 3: 211.

Luterkort M, Presson PH, Weldner BM. Maternal and fetal factors in breech presentations. *Obstet Gynecol* 1984; 64: 55.

Lydon-Rochelle M, Albers L, Gorwoda J, Craig E, Qualls C. Accuracy of Leopold manoeuvres in screening for malpresentation: a prospective study. *Birth* 1993; 20: 132.

Miller ME. Structural defects as a consequence of early intrauterine constraint: limb deficiency, polydactyly and body wall defects. *Semin Perinatol* 1983; 7: 277.

Miller ME, Dunn PM, Smith DW. Uterine malformation and fetal deformation. *J Pediatr* 1979; 94: 387.

Phillips CJ. *Hands of Love*. St Paul, Minnesota: New Dawn, 2001.

Pistolese RA. The Webster technique: a chiropractic with obstetric implications. *J Manipulative Physiol Ther* 2002; 25: E1–E9.

Sutton J, Scott P. *Optimal Foetal Positioning*. Tauranga, New Zealand: Birth Concepts, 1996.

Suzuki S, Yamamuro T. Fetal movement and fetal presentation. *Early Hum Dev* 1985; 11: 255.

Chiropractic Care During Pregnancy

Illustrations in Chapter One

Chapter 2
The birth process

The birth process and its natural physiological induction are complicated, so for the purpose of this book it will be covered briefly, and we will look in detail at aspects that have relevance to trauma to the infant and mother.

ENGAGEMENT

In the later weeks of pregnancy, the head often descends or engages as a precursor to the beginning of labour. Full engagement occurs when the biparietal diameter of the head (the widest point of the fetal skull) descends into the pelvic inlet (between the pubis and the sacral promontory). This is usually in the left occiput transverse position, i.e. the fetal occiput is on the left side of the maternal pelvis (Figure 2.1).

Synclitism and asynclitism

In a synclitic position, the sagittal suture lies along the transverse diameter of the pelvis (Figure 2.2). When the sagittal suture lies in any other position, it is termed asynclitism (Figure 2.3). A small amount of transitory asynclitism is generally seen in labour, and repeated movements of the fetal head may aid a

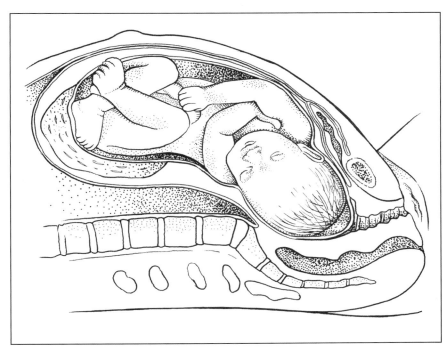

Figure 2.1 Full engagement of the fetal head.

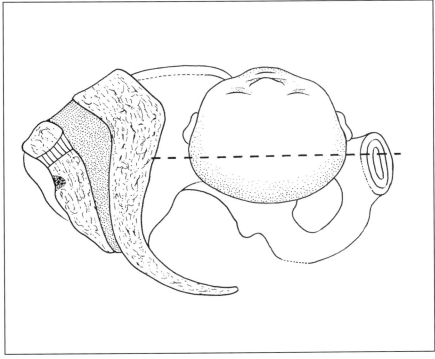

Figure 2.2 Synclitism. Adapted from Carrerio: An Osteopathic Approach to Children.

23

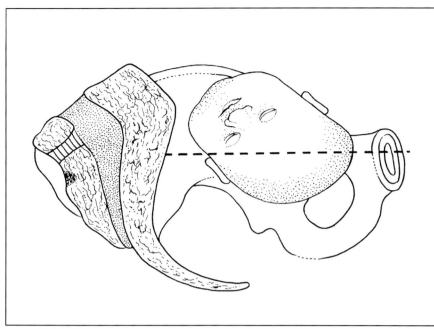

Figure 2.3 Asynclitism. Adapted from Carrerio: An Osteopathic Approach to Children.

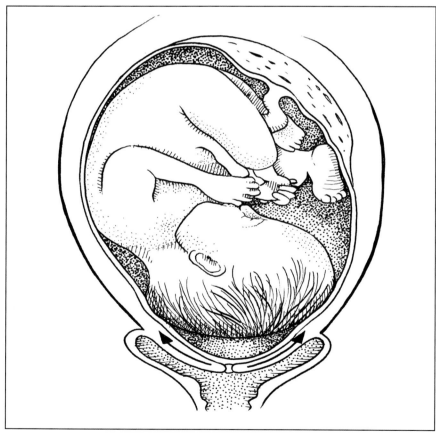

Figure 2.4 Effacement of the cervix.

smooth passage down the birth canal (Cunningham et al 2001)). However, if the head remains in an asynclitic position, this may interfere with normal rotation during descent and strain the tissues of the skull base (Carriero 2003).

STAGES OF LABOUR

There are four stages of labour:

- First stage – dilation of the cervix and upper birth canal.
- Second stage – expulsion of the fetus.
- Third stage – expulsion of the placenta.
- Fourth stage – early recovery.

For the purpose of this book, I will concentrate on the first two stages.

First stage of labour

The first stage of labour has two phases. Initially, there is a latent phase of 0–2.5 cm cervical dilatation, the average time for this being about 7.1 hours (Cunningham et al 2001). The woman is often unaware that she is in labour as the contractions can imitate the Braxton–Hicks contractions, which begin about 4 weeks prior to delivery and thin the lower uterine segment. Second, the active phase of the first stage occurs from 2.5 cm to full (10 cm) dilatation. This is marked by strong contractions and averages about 3.5 hours in length.

Each uterine contraction begins at the fundus and spreads towards the lower segment. During a contraction, the individual muscle fibres shorten. They then lengthen but not quite to their original length, remaining permanently shortened by a small amount; this is termed retraction. This means that the muscular fundus becomes thicker at the expense of the lower uterine segment, which becomes thinned and is taken up, or effaced (Quixley and Cameron 1979; Figure 2.4).

As labour progresses, the increasing strength of the uterine contractions pushes the presenting part of the fetus into the uterine fundus, expanding and dilating the cervix and stretching the pelvic soft tissues.

The cervix is effaced by the 'ball-valve' action of the fetal head on the forewaters (Figure 2.5). These forewaters are also protective of the fetal head, spreading out the force of the contractions. Amniotomy, one of the most common procedures in obstetrics, artificially ruptures the membranes, usually at about 5 cm dilatation, in order to speed up labour. This it very often does, but it also has the effect of increasing the stresses on the fetal head.

During descent, flexion of the fetus increases in response to the resistance of the maternal soft tissues. Fetal flexion is important as it protects the cervical spine. The cervical vertebrae stack up on their discs to provide protection to the posterior elements, particularly the nerve roots. The flexion of the fetal chin upon the chest helps to shift the head from the left occiput transverse to the left occiput anterior position.

Rotation

At the mid-pelvis, the head rotates 45 degrees to the right, turning the sagittal suture from a right oblique position to an anterior–posterior position (Figure 2.6). The shoulders of the

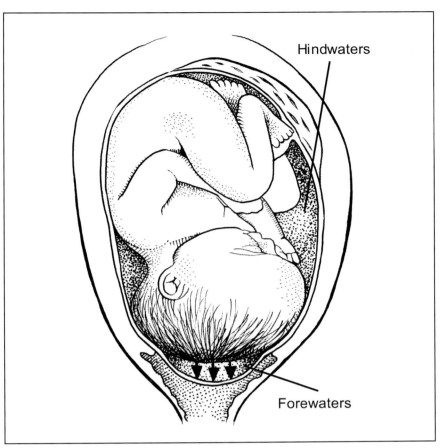

Figure 2.5 'Ball-valve' action of the fetal head.

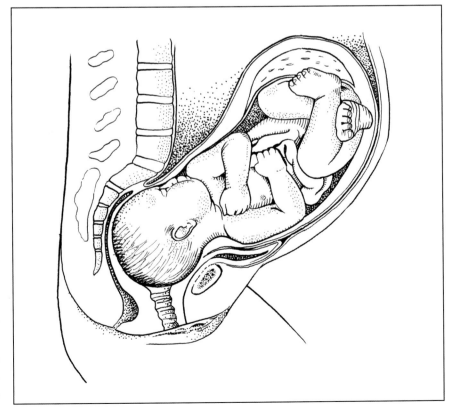

Figure 2.6 Internal rotation.

fetus remain in a left oblique position, this relationship persisting until delivery of the baby's head. As Carriero (2003) comments, one can immediately see the potential for tissue strain during prolonged deliveries.

Second stage of labour

The second stage begins at 10 cm dilatation, by which point the membranes have usually ruptured and contractions are occurring every 2–3 minutes. There are two phases to the second stage of labour.

During the first phase, there is little vaginal stretching, so no urge to bear down is present, but there may be some abdominal tightening as the fetal head descends. Phase 1 may be very short. Phase 2 begins when the mother gets to urge to bear down, greatly accelerating the passage of the fetus down the vagina. Delivery takes place on average in 10 contractions in muligravidae and 20 contractions in primagravidae (Cunningham et al 2001), but this can vary widely.

When the occiput has emerged from under the pubic symphysis and no longer slips back into the vagina, the head is said to have crowned. The head now slowly extends with the occiput pivoting on the pubic symphysis. The forehead and face are swept along the sacrum until the chin appears. The head then rotates to a neutral position with respect to the cervical spine, and the occiput is directed laterally. The head is now guided backwards to allow delivery of the anterior shoulder and then forwards to allow delivery of the posterior shoulder; the rest of the baby follows.

Cranial moulding

The cranium of the fetus moulds to allow it to accommodate to the shape of the birth canal. The frontal and occipital bones 'telescope' under the parietal bones, and the parietal bones themselves 'lock' together at the sagittal suture (Carlan et al 1991). This locking of the parietal bones probably protects the infant's brain and prevents excessive moulding and subsequent neurological damage. The suboccipito-bregmatic diameter shortens to about 9.5 cm to pass through the pelvis (Quixley and Cameron 1979), and the mento-vertical diameter lengthens (Figure 2.7). This occurs as the squamous occiput and the apexes of the two frontal bones move inwards using their basal portions as a hinge (Carlan et al 1991).

Arbuckle (1994) stated that the dura had a protective function in preventing excessive cranial moulding owing to the stress bands within the membranes. In other words, excessive compression of the brain would be resisted by particular bands of fibres within the reciprocal tension membranes. Arbuckle also suggested that when the skull base was distorted, these membranes would carry that distortion to the vault.

Moulding should normalise within 24 hours of birth, and the infant head regains its shape. Moulding that persists for

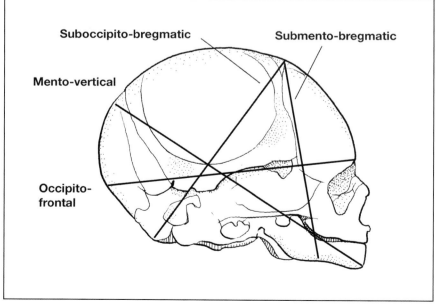

Figure 2.7 Fetal head diameters.

longer than this is an indication for cranial examination and care (Upledger 1996).

Rempen and Kraus (1991) measured fetal head pressures during delivery and found a wide variation in their readings. They noted that, during bearing down, there was higher pressure on the anterior side of the skull in comparison to the posterior side (maternal anterior–posterior). This is probably explained by the curved anatomy of the birth canal. It may have clinical relevance with a fetus that is stuck during descent, creating an uneven sheer stress to the cranial base. Rempen (1993) noted that fetal head pressure was higher in primiparae (probably owing to increased tissue resistance in the birth canal) and that oxytocin infusion significantly increased head pressure.

Vertical pressures during contractions are translated through the neonate along a cephalocaudal axis. Carreiro (2003) stated that these forces were primarily absorbed in the cranial base and vertebral column. The vertical forces travelling through the cranium meet resistance at the occipito-atlantal junction, which is usually locked in flexion. This is easier to deal with when the head is in a synclitic position as rotational and side-bending forces are not easily dealt with at the occipito-atlantal junction. The condyles, cranial base and vault take the stress if the head is fixed in an asynclitic position, and if descent is prevented by, for example, an anterior sacral base, strains of the skull base are likely.

The fetus is also susceptible to trauma during descent, when the head internally rotates 45 degrees (Figure 2.6 above). This rotation occurs when the fetal head comes up against the resistance of the true pelvis. The majority of the rotation occurs as would be expected between the atlas and axis, but some accommodation occurs at the next junctional area – the cervico-thoracic junction. According to Carriero (2003), flexion at the thoracic inlet and compressive forces on the rib cage limit the ability of the first thoracic vertebra to respond to this rotation so the forces are dispersed into the clavicles. Applied clinically, this tells us to examine carefully the clavicles and shoulders of neonates who have been stuck for an excessive time during descent. Cervico-thoracic, acromioclavicular, sternoclavicular and glenohumeral lesions are common. All the spinal junctional areas (upper cervical, cervico-thoracic, thoraco-lumbar and lumbo-sacral) are susceptible to rotational stress so need to be carefully assessed.

The next potential stress point the fetus may encounter is delivery of the head through the perineum. The occiput acts as a fulcrum for the extension of the head against the pubic symphysis so it is preferable for this stage to occur in a controlled fashion. The extension forces are transmitted primarily to the atlas, axis and occipital condyles and the occipital squama.

BIRTH TRAUMA

Major birth injuries are usually easily evidenced and so receive early diagnosis and treatment. Such injuries include fractures, brachial plexus lesions, lacerations, organ ruptures, dislocations and facial and other nerve lesions. I have found several undiagnosed clavicular fractures, congenital hip dislocations and cranial nerve palsies, so a thorough examination at first consultation is vital.

The majority of injuries dealt with in chiropractic clinics will, however, fall into the realm of more minor birth trauma, which often remains undiagnosed, and the parents are left with an apparently 'healthy' but unhappy baby. Gottlieb (1993, p 537), in an extensive literature review, stated that 'birth trauma is an under publicised and therefore untreated problem'. My experience suggests that Gottlieb's assertion is correct and that there is a growing epidemic of minor birth trauma, probably aggravated by the effect of the modern lifestyle on the female body (as described in Chapter 1) and the increased levels of intervention in the birth process currently seen.

Predisposing factors for birth trauma (Perlow et al 1996) include:

- the use of oxytocin;
- malpresentation;
- multiple pregnancy;
- prolonged labour;
- a prolonged second stage of labour;
- epidural anaesthesia;
- instrumental delivery;
- shoulder dystocia;
- macrosomia.

The causes of birth trauma can be divided into three broad groups:

1. intrauterine;
2. those occasioned during delivery;
3. iatrogenic.

This is, however, an artificial division because there is often a cascade of events taking one fetus through all three divisions. Using these divisions, however, simplifies the task of making sense of the events.

Intrauterine causes

Intrauterine constraint is stressful for the fetus and is a major cause of a dystocia and trauma to the neonate.

Breech presentation

Breech presentation (Figure 2.8) is a recognised risk factor for neonatal hip instability (Szepesi et al 1993). Sival et al (1993) found that breech-presenting infants had less hip extension and showed an abnormally flexed walking pattern at 12–18 months of age. Those breech presentations that proceed to a vaginal birth are also associated with high rates of genital oedema and ecchymosis. Carreiro (2003) comments that as the vertical compressive forces are increased in labour, the ischial tuberosities are forced medially and the sacrum inferiorly, into counternutation, which has the effect of flattening the lumbar spine. In the West, most breech presentations are currently delivered by elective caesarean section so hip instability and plagiocephaly are the main problems to be aware of.

Transverse lie

Transverse lies are indications for caesarean section if they fail to convert to a vertex presentation. Major causative factors are poor abdominal tone and high parity. They are associated with many neonatal deformities including plagiocephaly, torticollis, nasal septum deviation and foot deformities (Rossegger and Steinwender 1992).

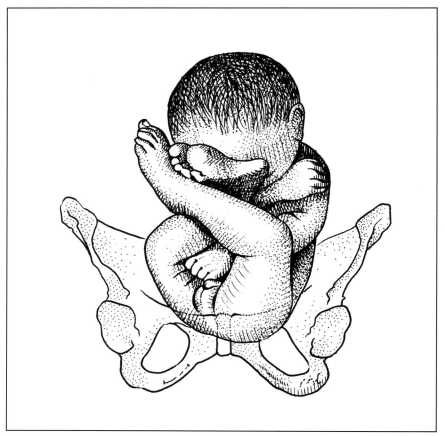

Figure 2.8 Frank breech presentation.

Multiple pregnancy

Twins have high rates of structural defects, mainly because of constraint. The most common examples are hip dysplasia, talipes and plagiocephaly (Cunningham et al 2001). In my experience regarding vaginal birth, the second-born twin often shows greater evidence of constraint and trauma than the first-born. Peitsch et al (2002) found an incidence of localised cranial flattening (often a precursor to deformational plagiocephaly) of 56% in infant twins examined.

Poor maternal condition

High parity and a lax abdominal wall are causes of malpresentation. In Chapter 1, it was stated that poor condition of the maternal abdominal and pelvic musculature might well have a wider relevance for fetal presentation and dystocia.

Genetic factors

Andrews and Jones (1998) found that anomalies of uterine structure were associated with preterm delivery, breech presentation, dysfunctional labour and operative delivery. Miller et al (1979) noted that fetal malformations, including hip dysplasia and plagiocephaly, were associated with uterine structural abnormalities.

DELIVERY

Prolonged labour

Dystocia means difficult labour and is characterised by an abnormally slow progress of labour. A prolonged second stage (which is in itself often associated with other interventions) is associated with clavicular fracture, facial nerve injury and brachial plexus injury (Perlow et al 1996).

A prolonged second stage is also, in my experience, a regular precursor to babies presenting at chiropractic clinics with a variety of symptoms usually resulting from occipital condylar compression.

Precipitate labour

Precipitate labour is expulsion of the fetus in less than 3 hours (Hughes 1972) and comprises approximately 2% of live births (Ventura et al 2000). It is associated with placental abruption (20%), postpartum haemorrhage and low Apgar scores (Mahon et al 1994). Some of the most symptomatically challenged infants I have encountered have undergone a precipitate labour and birth. Problems may result from excessively rapid cranial moulding, creating stress on the dura and therefore the nervous system.

Supine delivery

Supine delivery decreases the sagittal diameter of the birth canal by up to 1.5 cm because of the difficulty the sacrum has in rotating backwards. A randomised controlled trial by Gardosi et al (1989) of squatting in the second stage of labour found that this was associated with fewer forceps deliveries (9% versus 16%), a shorter second stage (31 versus 45 minutes) and fewer perineal but more labial tears.

Brow and face presentations

Both brow and face presentations result in hyperextension of the upper cervical spine and subsequent stress on the condylar portions of the occiput. Brow presentations are unstable and usually convert during labour to vertex or face. Face presentations can be delivered vaginally but are particularly compromised in a mentum posterior position, in which the bregma can become jammed against the pubic symphysis (Figure 2.9). Most neonates delivered from a face presentation exhibit significant facial oedema and bruising (Figure 2.10).

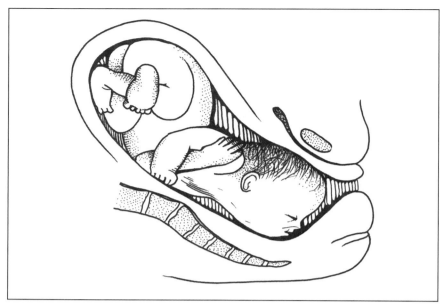

Figure 2.9 Face presentation.

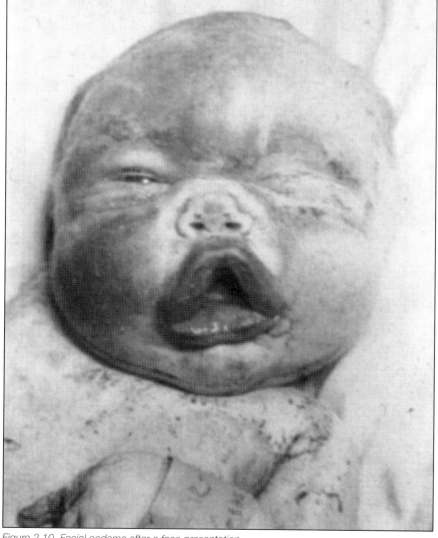

Figure 2.10 Facial oedema after a face presentation.

Persistent occiput posterior and occiput transverse presentations

These presentations are significant causes of dystocia and operative delivery if they do not rotate to occiput anterior (Fan et al 1997). Two large Chinese studies (Ox et al 1997, Wu et al 2001) have demonstrated the efficacy of the mother lying on the same side as the fetal spine during labour to correct persistent occiput posterior and transverse presentations: the rate of caesarean section decreased from 83.3% in the control group to 11.7% in the trial groups. Fetal hypoxia and neonatal asphyxia were also significantly more common in the abnormal occiput group.

Pregnant patients should be advised to lie on the same side as the fetal spine in the last few weeks of pregnancy to help prevent these presentations.

Induction

Labour is usually induced at about 42 weeks if it has not occurred spontaneously. Induction is also used when labour needs to be brought on early for such conditions as placental insufficiency and pre-eclampsia. Induction is associated with an increase in the rate of caesarean birth and other complications (Cunningham et al 2001).

Induction usually begins with an application of prostaglandin E2 gel to ripen the cervix, which is in some cases enough to start labour. This is often followed by intravenous oxytocin, which is a potent stimulant of uterine contractions. Oxytocin is associated with increased fetal head pressure (Rempen 1993) and operative delivery.

Membrane stripping – inserting a finger through the os and stripping away the membrane attachments – is relatively common practice to stimulate labour, particularly in the USA.

Amniotomy, or artificial rupture of the membranes, is among the most commonly performed procedures in obstetrics (Cunningham et al 2001). It is usually performed at around 5 cm dilatation and often speeds labour. As mentioned above, it does, however, remove the protective, cushioning effect of the forewaters and, combined with oxytocin infusion, will significantly increase fetal head pressure.

Operative delivery

Forceps are regularly used to assist delivery when there is a prolonged second stage of labour.

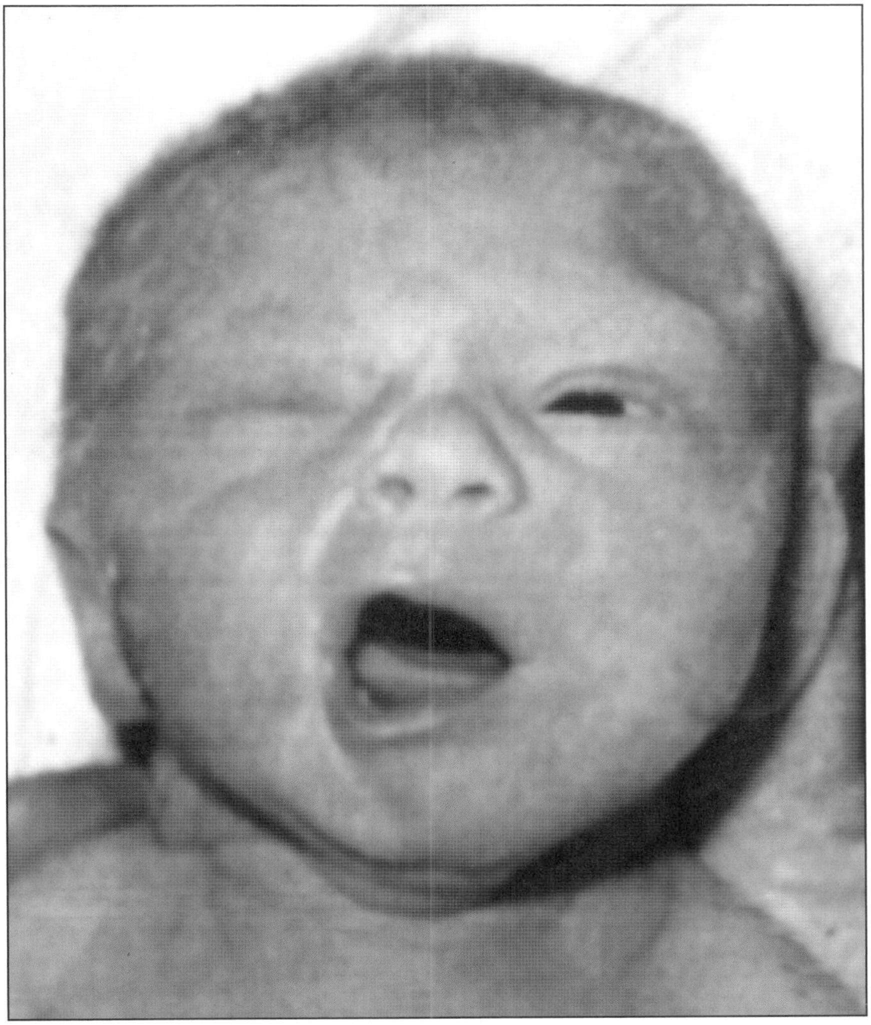

Figure 2.11 Facial nerve injury following forceps delivery.

Other indications are maternal health problems, cord prolapse, placental separation and fetal distress (American College of Obstetrics and Gynaecologists 2000).

Gardella et al (2001) commented that forceps delivery is associated with facial nerve injury (Figure 2.11), brachial plexus injury and intraventricular haemorrhage. Mid or rotational forceps deliveries demonstrate significantly increased levels of trauma compared with outlet forceps.

Interestingly, the long-term consequences of forceps delivery include higher percentages of adult bruxism, temporomandibular joint crepitus and pain (Germane and Rubenstein 1989) and asymmetrical occlusions (Pirttiniemi et al 1994). A high rate of anal sphincter incompetence (32%) is one of the long-term consequences for the woman who has a child delivered by forceps (Sultan et al 1996).

Vacuum extraction has been in wide usage since the 1950s. It has been linked to higher levels of cephalhaematoma, jaundice, intercranial haemorrhage and shoulder dystocia (Gardella et al 2001, Shihadeh and Al- Najdawi 2001). Carriero (2003) notes a helicoidal tissue strain pattern in the crania of infants after vacuum extraction.

Deliveries via caesarean section are becoming more common: according to Cunningham et al

31

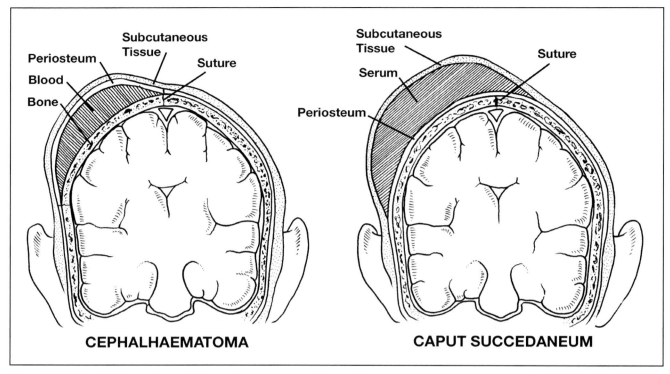

Figure 2.12 Differential diagnosis – cephalhaematoma versus caput succendaneum.

(2001), they now make up 25% of recorded births in the USA. There are significant differences in the trauma levels and symptomatology of infants born by caesarean section in labour or electively. Caesarean section in labour is often the end of the line following other failed attempts at operative intervention and is often an emergency procedure in response to fetal distress. Infants born by elective section do not have the trauma of failed labour to stress their systems. Although infants delivered by elective section have a low level of birth trauma, it is likely that some of the reflex stimulatory effect of delivery through the birth canal is lost.

Caput succedaneum and cephalhaematoma

Many infants present after traumatic deliveries with swelling of the cranium. The differential diagnosis is important for the prognosis of the swelling and for contraindications to cranial adjusting.

Caput succedaneum (Figure 1.12) is a diffuse soft tissue swelling consisting of lymph and blood lying under the subcutaneous tissue; this will often resolve in days. The swelling will often cross suture lines as it is located above the periosteum of the skull.

Cephalhaematoma (Figure 2.12) is a subperiosteal bleed, which does not cross suture lines and may take weeks to resolve. Some ossify and become permanent skull distortions. Cephalhaematomas have an association with skull fractures (Cunningham et al 2001) and as such must be regarded as at least a caution when undertaking cranial work in the first 8 weeks of life.

REFERENCES

American College of Obstetricians and Gynecologists. Operative Vaginal Delivery. *Practice Bulletin No. 17*. Washington: ACOG, 2000.

Andrews MC, Jones HW. Impaired human reproductive performance of unicornate uterus: intra uterine growth retardation, infertility and recurrent abortion. *Am J Obstet Gynecol* 1998; 19: 939.

Arbuckle BE. *The Selected Works of Beryl E Arbuckle*. Indianapolis: American Academy of Osteopathy, 1994.

Carlan SJ, Wyble L, Lense J, Mastrogiannis DS, Parsons MT. Fetal head moulding. Diagnosis by ultrasound and a review of the literature. *J Perinatal* 1991; 11: 105–111.

Carreiro JE. An *Osteopathic Approach to Children*. Edinburgh: Churchill Livingstone, 2003.

Cunningham GF, Gant NF, Leveno KJ, Gilstrap LC, Hauth JC, Wenstrom KD. *Williams' Obstetrics, 21st edn*. New York: McGraw-Hill, 2001.

Fan L, Huang X, Wang Q. The characteristics of labour course and perinatal prognosis in cases of fetal persistent occiput – transverse and persistent occiput – posterior position. *Zhonghua Fu Chan Ke Za Zhi* 1997; 32: 620–622.

Gardella C Taylor M, Benedetti T, Hitti J, Critchlow C. The effect of sequential use of vacuum and forceps for assisted vaginal delivery on neonatal and maternal outcomes. *Am J Obstet Gynecol* 2001;185: 896–902.

Gardosi J, Hutson N, Lynch CB. Randomised controlled trial of squatting in the second stage of labour. *Lancet* 1989; July: 74–77.

Germane N, Rubenstein L. The effects of forceps on facial growth. *Pediatr Dent* 1989; 11: 193.

Gottlieb MS. Neglected spinal cord, brain stem and musculoskeletal injuries stemming from birth trauma. *J Manipulative Physiol Ther* 1993; 16: 537–543.

Hughes EC. *Obstetric–Gynecologic Terminology*. Philadelphia: FA Davis, 1972.

Mahon TR, Chazotte C, Cohen WR. Short labor: characteristics and outcome. *Obstet Gynecol* 1994; 84: 47–51.

Miller ME, Dunn PM, Smith DW. Uterine malformation and fetal deformation. *J Pediatr* 1979; 94: 387.

Ou X, Chen X, Su J. Correction of occiput posterior position by maternal posture during the process of labor. *Zhonghua Fu Chan Ke Za Zhi* 1997: 32: 329.

Peitsch WK, Keefer CH, LaBrie RA, Mulliken JB. Incidence of cranial asymmetry in healthy newborns. *Pediatrics* 2002;110: e72.

Perlow JH, Wigton T, Hart J, Strassner HT, Nageotte MP, Wolk BM. Birth trauma. A five year review of incidence and associated perinatal factors. *J Reprod Med* 1996; 41: 754–760.

Pirttiniemi P, Gron M, Alvesalo L, Heikkinen T, Osborne R. Relationship of difficult forceps delivery to dental arches and occlusion. *Pediatr Dent* 1994; 16: 289.

Quixley JME, Cameron MD. *Obstetrics and Gynaecology, 4th edn*. London: Hodder & Stoughton, 1979.

Rempen A. Stress on the head of the fetus in spontaneous labor in relation to perinatal factors. *Z Geburtshilfe Perinatol* 1993; 197: 77–83.

Rempen A, Kraus M Pressures on the fetal head during normal labor. *J Perinat Med* 1991; 19: 199–206.

Rosseger H, Steinwender G. Transverse fetal position syndrome – a combination of skeletal deformities in the new born infant. *Padiatr Padol* 1992; 27: 125–127.

Shihadeh A, Al-Najdawi W. Forceps or vacuum extraction: a comparison of maternal and neonatal morbidity. *East Mediterr Health J* 2001; 7: 106–114.

Sival DA, Prechtl HF, Sonder GH, Touwen BC. The effect of intra-uterine breech position on postnatal motor functions of the lower limbs. *Early Hum Dev* 1993; 32: 161–176.

The birth process

Sultan AH, Stanton SL. Preserving the pelvic floor and perineum during childbirth: elective caesarean section? Br *J Obstet Gynaecol* 1996; 103: 731.

Szepesi J, Hattyar A, Molnar L. The effect of breech presentation on the development of the hips. *Magy Traumatol Ortop Kezeb Plasztikai Seb* 1993; 36: 11–15.

Upledger JE. *A Brain Is Born.* Berkley: North Atlantic Books, 1996.

Ventura SJ, Martin JA, Curtin SC, Matthews TJ, Park MM. Births: Final Data for 1998. *National Vital Statistics Reports, Vol. 28*, No. 3. Hyattsville, Maryland: National Centre for Health Statistics, 2000.

Wu X, Fan L, Wang Q. Correction of occiput posterior by maternal postures during the process of labor. *Zhonghua Fu Chan Ke Za Zhi* 2001; 36: 468.

Illustrations in Chapter Two

Chapter 3
Neonatal and infant examination

HISTORY

An accurate prenatal and natal history is an essential precursor to a thorough and complete examination. It is also a useful time in establishing a rapport with the parent(s).

Prenatal history

- What was the mother's health status before and during pregnancy?

- What was her age?

- Was it her first pregnancy?

- What was her history of drug (prescription or otherwise) and alcohol use during and before the pregnancy?

- How much weight did she gain in pregnancy?

- Were there any complications or problems with the pregnancy?

- How many weeks gestation was the pregnancy?

- Do the parents have any concerns about the pregnancy or the birth?

Natal history

The birth history is obviously very important, but the parents are often unable to give a full account so specific questions and some reading between the lines is often necessary to find out what happened during the birth.

- What drugs if any were used?

- Was the birth spontaneous or induced?

- Was instrumentation (i.e. forceps or vacuum extraction) used?

- Were the membranes artificially ruptured?

- Was an episiotomy performed?

- What position did the mother labour and give birth in?

- What position was the fetus in the second stage (occiput posterior, occiput transverse, breech, etc.)?

- Did the mother think that the birth was excessively traumatic?

- Where did the birth take place – at home, in hospital or elsewhere?

Neonatal history

- Was the child given directly to the mother following birth or was resuscitation necessary?

- What were the infant's Apgar scores?

- Was the infant wakeful and responsive?

- Did the infant feed spontaneously?

- Was there jaundice present?

- What was the mother's health status postpartum?

Apgar score

The Apgar score is a method of assessing the infant's systemic response to birth and reflects the stress experienced by the neonate during the birth process. It is assessed at 1 and 5 minutes after birth. Five variables are assessed – heart rate, respiratory effort, muscle tone, reflex irritability and colour – and are assigned numerical values between 0 and 2. This recording serves two purposes. First, it ensures a careful evaluation of the newborn, and second, it helps to determine the presence of central nervous system depression and whether there is a need for resuscitation.

A low Apgar score does not necessarily mean that the infant is suffering from asphyxia, as was previously thought. Low Apgar scores may be caused by many conditions, such as sepsis and neuromuscular disorders, as well as perinatal asphyxia Compression of the fetal head may result in a decreased heart rate (Mocsary et al 1970).

Gestational age and neonatal size are important factors in the health of the newborn infant. Term infants are those with a gestational age between 38 and 42 weeks, preterm those born

Neonatal and infant examination

	0	1	2	3	4	5
Skin	Gelatinous, red, transparent	Smooth, pink, visible veins	Superficial peeling and/ or rash, few veins	Cracking, pale areas, rare veins	Parchment, deep cracking, no vessels	Leathery, cracked, wrinkled
Lanugo	None	Abundant	Thinning	Bald areas	Mostly bald	
Plantar creases	No crease	Faint red marks	Anterior transverse crease only	Creases anterior two thirds	Creases cover entire sole	
Breast	Barely perceptible	Flat areola, no bud	Stippled areola, 1-2mm bud	Raised areola, 3-4mm bud	Full areola 5-10mm bud	
Ear	Pinna flat, stays folded	Pinna slightly curved, soft, slow recoil	Well curved pinna, soft but steady recoil	Formed and firm with instant recoil	Thick cartilage, ear stiff	
Male genitals	Scrotum empty, no rugae		Testes descending, few rugae	Testes down, good rugae	Testes pendulous deep rugae	
Female genitals	Prominent clitoris and labia minora		Majora and minora equally prominent	Majora large, minora small	Clitoris and minora completely covered	

Maturity rating

Score	Weeks
5	26
10	28
15	30
20	32
25	34
30	36
35	38
40	40
45	42
50	44

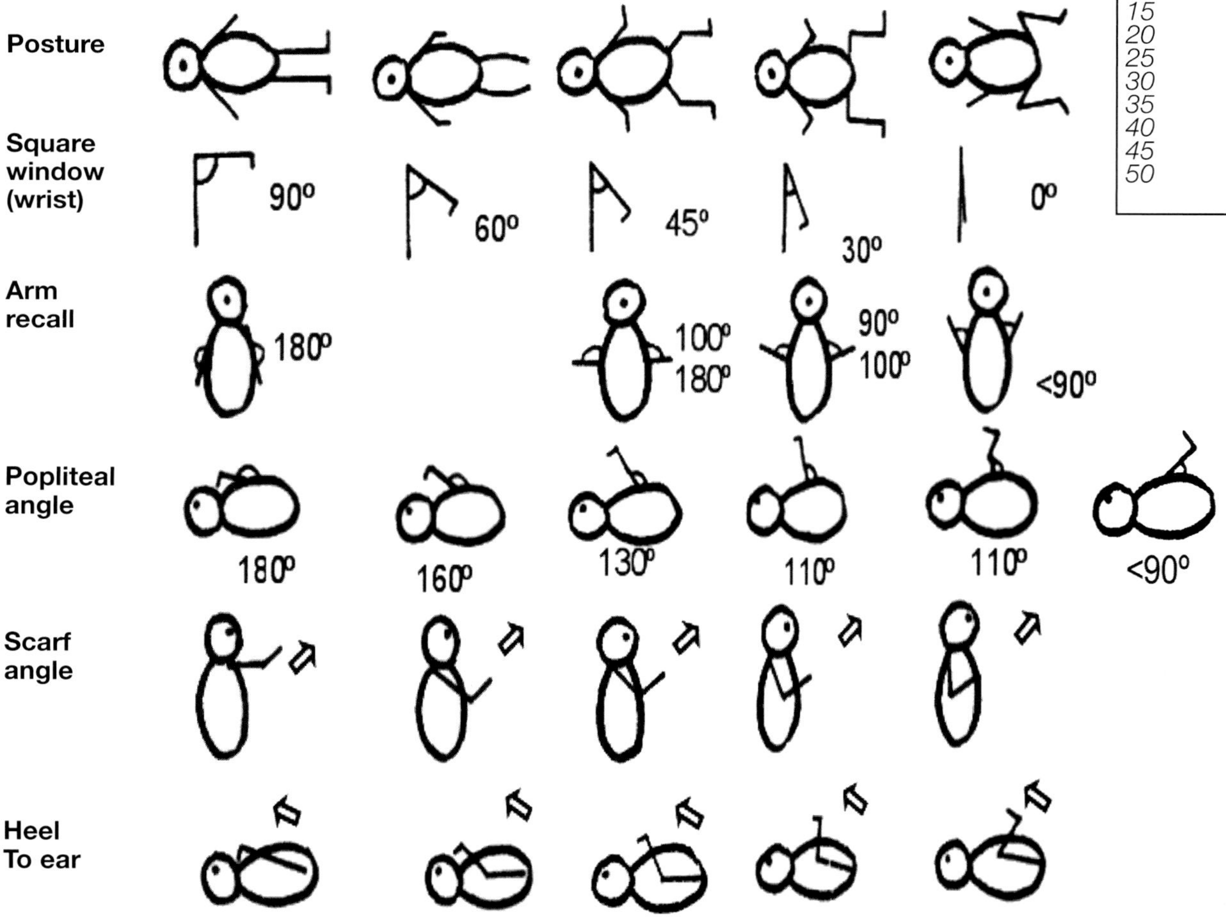

Figure 3.1 Chart for assessing gestational maturity (from Ballard et al 1979).

36

prior to 38 weeks and post-term those born after 42 weeks. The most reliable and accurate way to assess gestational age is, however, using the infant's physical cha-racteristics and neuromuscular abilities (Figure 3.1).

History of infancy

- Was the child breast-fed or bottle-fed, or were both given?

- Did the infant have a tendency when sitting or lying to hold his or her head in lateral flexion or extension?

- Were there any problems with feeding (i.e. posseting, not latching on, not feeding as well from one or other breast, abdominal colic, constipation or diarrhoea)?

- At what age was the child weaned, and which foodstuffs were used?

- What is the infant's sleep pattern?

- At what age did the infant gain head control, sit up, roll over, walk, etc.?

EXAMINATION OF THE NEONATE AND YOUNG INFANT

Most chiropractors do not work in the obstetric or immediate neonatal primary care area: we generally see our young patients after they have returned home from the birth centre and have undergone their initial checks with the medical doctors. It is

easy to assume that these are full and complete checks and that no significant damage or pathology will be present. This has not, however, been my experience, and over the years I have observed many hip instabilities, cranial nerve lesions, developmental delays and even a few fractures that have been missed. This is not to criticise those clinicians who performed the initial examinations, but rather to emphasise that the examination of neonates and infants is not easy and we all can miss things. There is no substitute for a thorough and detailed scrutiny of our little patients.

The ideal time to examine a newborn is a couple of hours after a feed, when the baby is not as deeply asleep as after a feed, and is not crying vigorously, as just before a feed. I have found it not to be a good idea to see infants at the end of the day's clinic: they are often irritable in the early evening.

The first thing to do is to observe: there is much we can learn from observation, and young infants often do not tolerate too much poking and prodding without showing irritation. When ob-serving the baby, the following questions should be asked:

- Does the baby look normal or abnormal?
- Is the baby in proportion?
- Are there any physical deformities or malformations?

- Is there any obvious respiratory effort? (Look for indrawing of the intercostal muscles and areas around the sternum.)
- Does the baby's skin appear to be well oxygenated and pink? (In darker-skinned races, check the palms, lips, conjunctivae and buccal mucosa.)

The cranium

Chapter 7 will deal in detail with the assessment and correction of cranial strain patterns. In newborns, moulding from the birth process is often present and can sometimes exhibit patterns related to the presentation of the baby (Figure 3.2). Excessive cranial moulding is of particular concern to the craniopath and can give rise to significant skull strain patterns that not only are of cosmetic concern, but may also, as we will see in later chapters, be associated with some significant health issues.

On initial examination of the cranium, it is obviously important to check for symmetry. This is undertaken from the anterior, looking at the levels of the eyes, ears and maxilla, noting any distortions, and from above, looking at the overall shape and the relative positions of the ears and nose. These factors give us guidance to the presence of any strain patterns. The presence of such factors as low-set ears and wide-set eyes can also alert the clinician to the possibility of the presence of genetic disorders such as Down's syndrome.

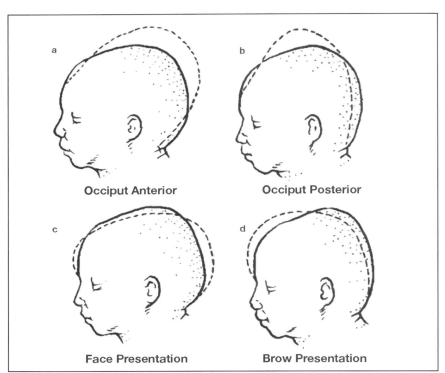

Figure 3.2 Cranial moulding according to fetal position: (a) left occiput anterior, (b) right occiput posterior, (c) facial presentation (full extension), and (d) brow presentation (partial extension). Adapted from Pediatric Chiropractic Anrig and Plaugher eds.

The skin

Gestational age can cause variations in the appearance of a newborn's skin, and full or post-dates babies can exhibit mild-to-moderate peeling.

Milia are common. This is a rash of white, pinhead-sized concretions, usually on the face. These are actually tiny sebaceous retention cysts and should disappear in the first few weeks of life.

Erythema toxicum is the name given to numerous small areas of red skin, often with a yellowish or whitish papule in the centre. They are commonly observed at around 2 days old and may last for 7–10 days.

Mongolian spots are common in black and Asian children around the back and trunk and can last up to 4 years. They resemble bruises and can be mistaken for signs of physical abuse.

'Stork marks' or *macular haemangiomas* are often seen around the occiput, forehead and eyes. They are supposed to be of little clinical significance, but in my opinion they show the areas of the cranium that underwent sustained pressure during the birth process.

A normal newborn's skin should be well oxygenated and pink; in babies from darker-skinned races, this pinkness is best observed on the palms, lips, buccal mucosa and conjunctivae. It is, however, common for newborns to exhibit *acrocyanosis* (a bluish or purplish tinge to the hands and feet). Any central cyanosis (tongue and lips), significant jaundice, plethora or petechial haemorrhages are abnormal and require referral for further investigation.

Some babies' extremities may show also a mottled pattern if they are cool; this is known as *cutis marmorata* or marble skin. It should be noted, however, that generalised mottling might signify acidosis or vascular instability.

An interesting colour change is present in the so-called *harlequin syndrome*, occasionally seen in low birthweight babies. This occurs where the upper half of the baby appears pale compared with the dark pink or reddish lower half, with a fairly sharp mid-section demarcation line. This unusual phenomenon has no pathological significance.

The cry

It is important to be able to recognise babies' normal cries, for example if they are tired or hungry or need changing. The cry should be strong; a low- or high-pitched cry or one exhibiting hoarseness or weakness can indicate laryngeal or neurological abnormalities. Hypothyroidism often shows as a low, throaty cry.

NEUROLOGICAL EXAMINATION OF THE NEWBORN

Position and muscle tone

A newborn baby should show a resting flexed posture. This means that, when the baby is lying supine, the hips, knees and elbows are generally held in slight flexion (Figure 3.3). A newborn who has spent some time in a distorted intrauterine position as a result of constraint may show that distortion pattern when observed lying supine. A note should be made of any body curves, head lateral flexion, rotation or extension and the position of the limbs. This can give a strong indication of where to look for fascial or joint restrictions.

Curvature of the infant's trunk can be due to rib subluxations and fascial tensions (be aware of the possibility of anomalies, e.g. hemivertebrae). Rotation/lateral flexion/extension of the head can be caused by upper cervical or occipital base lesions. Abnormal positioning of the limbs can be due to extremity subluxations, hip dysplasia or fascial torsion (be aware of the possibility of clavicular fractures – I have seen several in practice).

By watching the infant and flexing and extending their extremities, the clinician can gain an impression of the infant's resting tone, which is graded as normal,

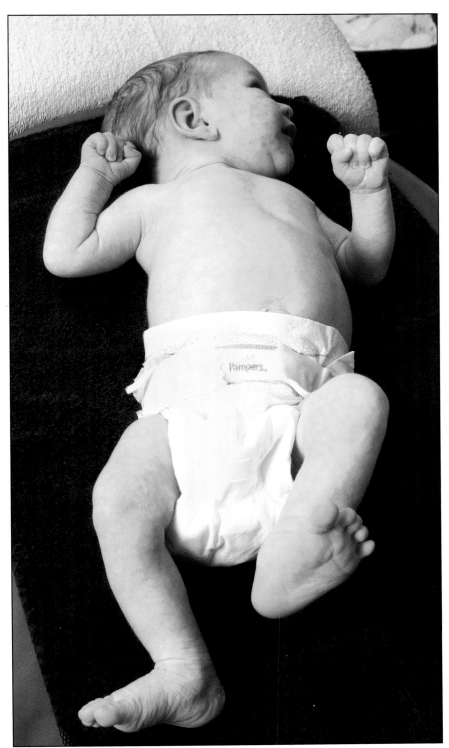

Figure 3.3 Resting flexed posture in a newborn.

increased or diminished (Figure 3.4). The differences one finds are difficult to describe in words, and only by making it a regular practice to move the limbs during examination of the infant will the

necessary expertise be gained and an instinctive feel for normal and abnormal developed.

When the newborn is pulled into the sitting position from supine, the head will lag behind

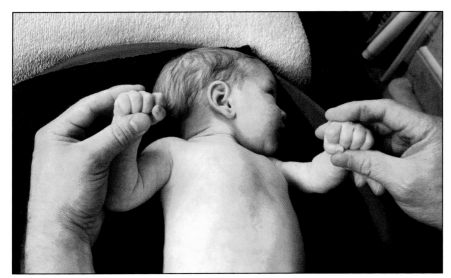

Figure 3.4 Assesment of tone in the extremities.

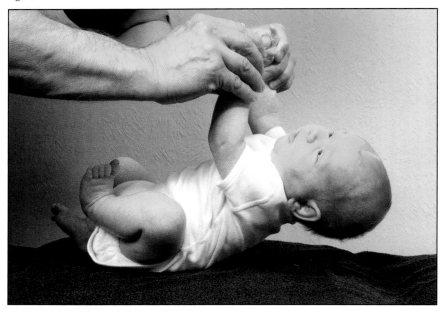

Figure 3.5 Head lag at 3 weeks of age.

hammer (Figure 3.6). The triceps reflex can sometimes be difficult to obtain because of flexor tone, but all the others should be brisk and symmetrical.

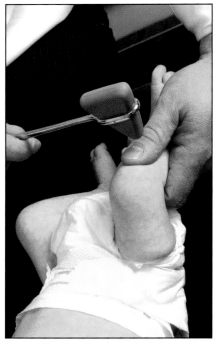

Figure 3.6 Deep tendon reflexes – patellar reflex.

the trunk. A healthy newborn will, however, make some effort to keep the head in line with the trunk, and once lifted into the sitting position, a healthy full term newborn should be able to keep his or her head upright for a few seconds (Figure 3.5). By 10 weeks of age, the infant's head will travel in line with the spine, and by 20–24 weeks, the head will lead the shoulders (Shumway-Cook and Woollacott 2000).

Lesions of the upper cervical spine and cranial base can contribute to hyper- or hypotonia in the newborn and should be examined and corrected as soon as possible.

Deep tendon reflexes

Deep tendon reflexes should be assessed in all neonatal examinations. This is best done by placing a finger over the tendon and striking it gently with a reflex

Extensor plantar (Babinski) response

The plantar surface of the foot is firmly stroked from the heel, along the lateral border and then crossing the metatarsals to the medial border. The extensor plantar response consists of extension of the great toe and flaring of the other four toes. This is considered normal up to 12 months of age and of equivocal clinical significance until the child is walking provided that is before 18 months of age. Asymmetry is, however, always considered abnormal, and other factors such as deep tendon reflex clonus and spasticity should be evaluated.

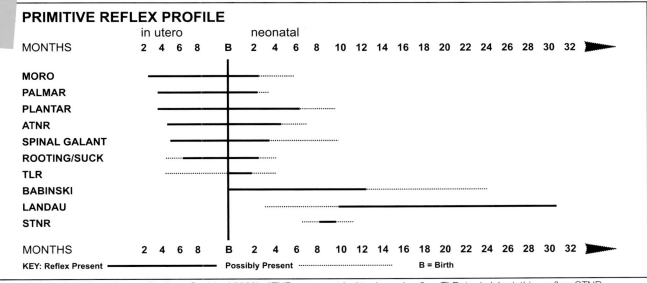

PRIMITIVE REFLEX PROFILE

Figure 3.7   Primitive reflex profile (from Goddard 2002). ATNR, asymmetrical tonic neck reflex; TLR, tonic labyrinthine reflex; STNR, symmetrical tonic neck reflex.

Primitive (neonatal) reflexes

Many of the so-called primitive reflexes develop in utero and are essential to the baby's survival in the first few weeks of life. They are automatic, stereotyped movements directed from the brainstem without cortical involvement and are inhibited by the development of postural reflexes at 6–12 months of age. If they remain active before this point, they are evidence of a structural weakness or immaturity within the central nervous system (Goddard 2002).

We shall look at reflex retention in relation to specific complaints later in this book.

It is thought that some of the primitive reflexes present in utero (e.g. spinal galant, asymmetrical tonic neck reflex) help the fetus in its journey into the world in 'wriggling' its way

down the birth canal. The length of time for which a reflex is present is variable (Figure 3.7). A primitive reflex evaluation provides us with information about both the musculoskeletal and neurological systems.

Moro, startle or embrace reflex

This reflex emerges in utero and should be beginning to be inhibited in its crude form by 4

months of age, to be replaced by an adult startle or Strauss reflex.

Newborns can demonstrate the Moro reflex spontaneously when suddenly moved, exposed to a loud noise or rapidly tipped backwards (Figure 3.8). The reflex is most easily demonstrated by letting the infant's head fall backwards (still lightly supported) below the level of the rest of the body while the baby is held supine. This will cause the

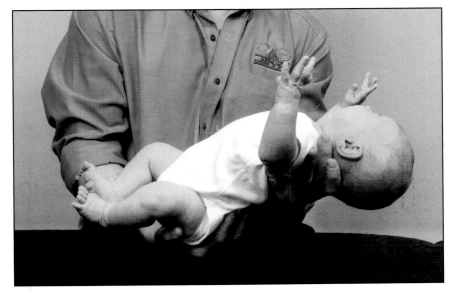

Figure 3.8 Moro response.

baby to extend his or her arms rapidly with the hands open and then bring them back more slowly into an embrace-type movement. This may well be accompanied by a grimace and a cry. Symmetry and movement are important – asymmetrical arm movement may result from clavicular fracture, brachial plexus injury or an extremity lesion.

A hyperactive Moro embrace, i.e. a baby who regularly startles with very little stimulation, can, in my experience, be a sign of severe compression or torsion of the sphenoid bone. These babies are often very unsettled, cry persistently and sleep little. A baby who regularly wakes screaming should be examined for the presence of sphenoid lesions.

The Moro reflex is the earliest form of the 'fight or flight' response and as such involves excitation of all the body systems involved in fight or flight. If it is not inhibited properly, it may result in hypersensitivity in one or several sensory systems, causing an overreaction to stimuli such as touch, noise and light, and leading to adrenal exhaustion, as is commonly seen in children with attention deficit hyperactivity disorder.

Palmar grasp reflex

This emerges in utero and is inhibited by 3 months of age.

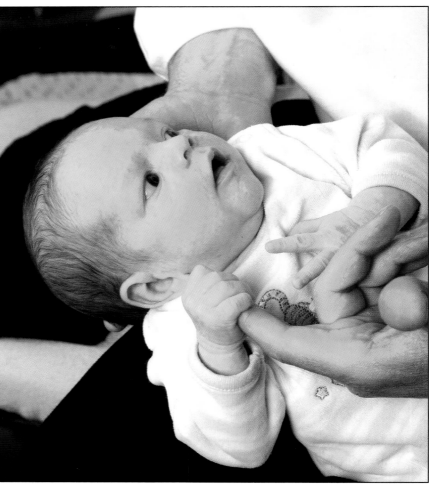

Figure 3.9 Palmar grasp reflex.

When a finger is placed in the baby's open hands, the baby's fingers should close around this and grip strongly enough to allow him or her to be lifted at least part way off the table (Figure 3.9). The palmar grasp can be elicited by the action of the baby sucking and may cause kneading of the hands in time with the sucking movements (Babkin response). It is thought the palmar reflex is an evolutionary hang-over from when our ancestors had to hang on to their mothers immediately after birth.

Retention of the palmar reflex beyond 4–5 months will impede manual dexterity and cause difficulties with such activities as handwriting. Speech may also be affected as a continuing relationship between mouth and hand movements will impede the development of muscular control at the front of the mouth (Goddard 2002).

Asymmetrical tonic neck reflex

This emerges in utero, to be inhibited by the time the baby is 6 months old.

To test for this reflex, the infant lies supine and the examiner rotates the head to one side looking for

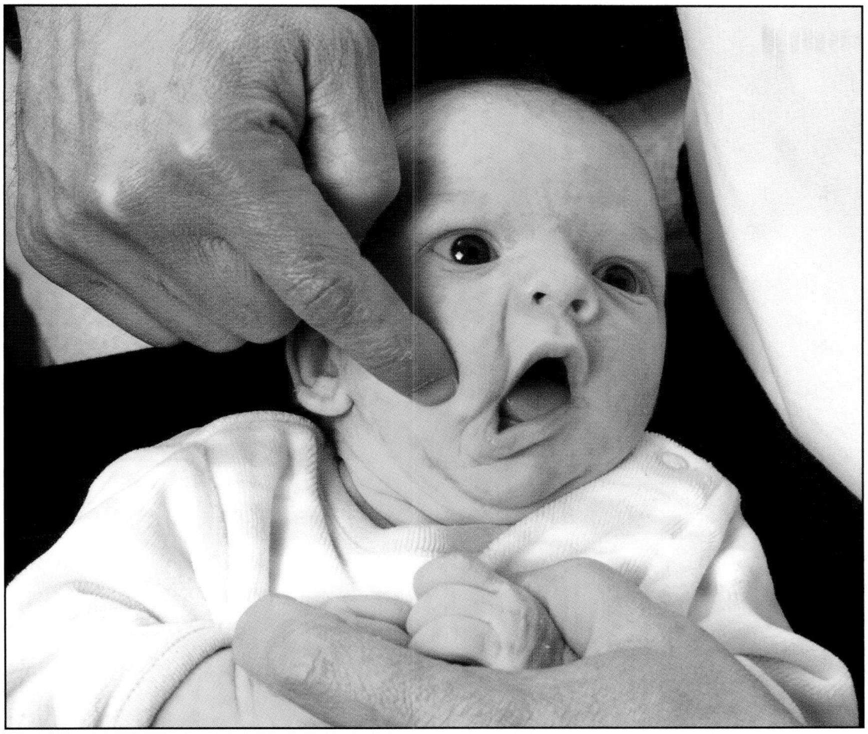

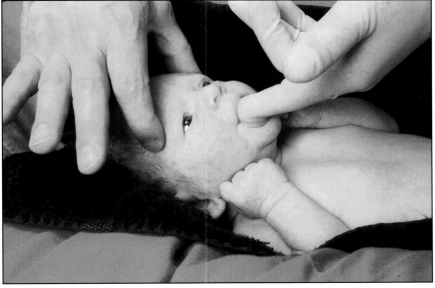

Figure 3.10 Rooting reflex.

Rooting reflex

The rooting reflex emerges in utero and is inhibited by 4 months old.

The reflex is initiated by stroking the baby's cheek from the lateral edge of the zygoma down to the chin. The infant's response should be a 'rooting' of the mouth towards the examiner's finger as if he or she is going to suck it (Figure 3.10). The reflex should be equal bilaterally. It is temporarily inhibited when the infant is satiated.

The rooting reflex can be an indicator of central nervous system function, but I have seen an inhibition of this reflex unilaterally and bilaterally in facial trauma (forceps deliveries and face presentations), which responded well to cranial adjustments. Retention of this reflex can lead to difficulty with solid foods and swallowing, and, later on, speech problems.

Suck reflex

The suck reflex has its onset in utero and is inhibited by 4 months old.

Figure 3.11 Suck reflex and sphenoid palpation.

extension of the upper and lower extremity on the ipsilateral side. The test is performed bilaterally. The body's response resembles a fencer's posture. Because of this response, it is important, when doing these tests, that the baby's head is in the midline. Asymmetry of the reflex can indicate hemiparesis, clavicular fracture, a brachial plexus lesion or a subluxation of the extremity. Retention of this reflex after 6 months of age will interfere with crawling and make it difficult for infants to manipulate objects from one hand to another across the midline.

This reflex, like the rooting reflex, is critical for spontaneous feeding. It is examined by placing a gloved finger in the baby's mouth. The finger should be drawn up and back towards the soft palate by the baby's sucking action (Figure 3.11). The tongue should also show a rippling motion along the finger as if it were stimulating the nipple to provide milk.

There are many types of suck and sucking disorders. Suffice it to say that the suck should be enthusiastic without being too strong – I have seen many mothers with cracked and painful nipples from an overly strong suck reflex. Although the suck response again to some extent illustrates central nervous system function, it is often inhibited by hypoglossal canal compression and, in my experience, becomes overactive when the maxillae are compressed.

Retention of the suck reflex can, as with the rooting reflex, lead to chewing, swallowing and speech problems.

Spinal galant (trunk incurvation) reflex

The spinal galant emerges in utero, to be inhibited at 3–8 months old.

The baby is tested prone and the paraspinal musculature stroked from the shoulder to sacrum. The baby should flex laterally and extend to the ipsilateral side (Figure 3.12). The reflex should be tested bilaterally.

This is a spinal cord reflex so its absence may be indicative of a cord lesion. Retention of this reflex is linked to fidgeting and bed-wetting. The latter is caused by bilateral stimulation of the reflex activating the Pulgar Marx reflex (which probably helps to

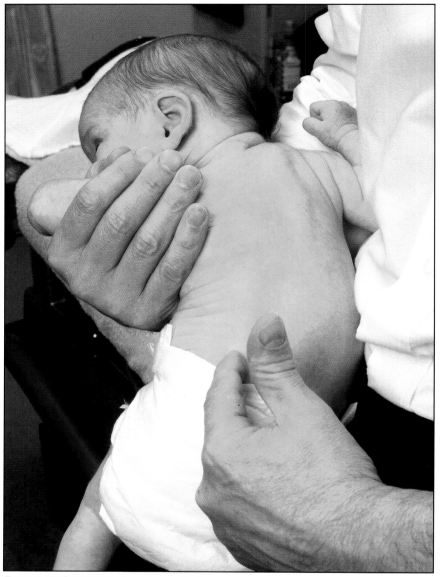

Figure 3.12 Galant's test (trunk incurvation).

decrease the infant's volume by voiding urine when it is stimulated bilaterally in the birth process by the walls of the birth canal) and leading to a voiding of urine. Retention of this reflex is also commonly found in a high percentage of people with irritable bowel syndrome (Goddard 2002).

Tonic labyrinthine reflex

The tonic labyrinthine reflex (TLR) forwards emerges at birth and is inhibited at 4 months of age. The TLR backwards emerges at birth and is inhibited in a gradual progression 6 weeks to 3 years old.

The TLR forwards is tested by flexing the head forwards, which leads to flexion of the baby's trunk and limbs (Figure 3.13). The TLR backwards is tested by extending the baby's neck, which leads to an extension of all four limbs. Both reflexes play a part in the birth process, the TLR forwards contributing towards the fetus's flexed position in utero and TLR backwards aiding in birth when the head extends after it has been delivered, leading to limb extension and allowing an easier delivery of the body.

Limb movements should be observed to be symmetrical. Lesions of the occipital condyles caused by extension in the birth process can lead to the infant becoming distressed on testing the TLR forwards. Retention of the TLR forwards can lead to a stooped posture, hypotonus and coordination and balance problems. Retention of the TLR backwards can lead to toe-walking, hypertonus and coordination problems.

Blink reflex

A bright light (a pen torch) is shone into the infant's eyes. This response assesses a limited level of visual activity, the normal response being a tight shutting of the eyes.

Acoustic blink

The acoustic blink emerges at birth and is inhibited with the Moro reflex.

The examiner claps his or her hands out of the infant's gaze; the infant should respond by blinking the eyes or may even show a full Moro response. To a limited degree, this tests auditory function.

Placing response

The placing response emerges at birth, being inhibited at about 2 months of age.

The examiner holds the baby upright and places the sole of one foot on the table. The baby's other leg is then drawn up as if he or she is about to walk (Figure 3.14) – parents love this! If the reflex is absent on one side, suspect a congenital

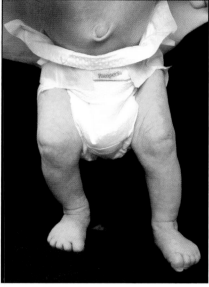

Figure 3.14 Placing response.

hip dysplasia or lower extremity subluxation.

Plantar grasp

The plantar grasp emerges in utero and is inhibited by 4 months old.

The examiner's thumb is placed on the sole of the baby's foot in the space under the toes; a strong grip response is normal (Figure 3.15).

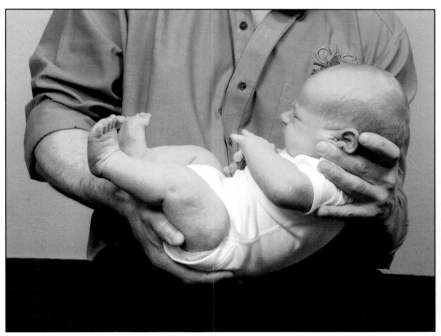

Figure 3.13 Tonic labyrinthine reflex forwards.

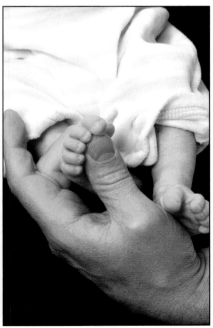

Figure 3.15 Plantar grasp.

Vertical suspension (Landau) reflex

The vertical suspension reflex emerges at birth, to be inhibited by 6 months old.

The examiner supports the infant around the torso and, with the infant upright, lifts the baby suddenly towards the ceiling. The response should be bilateral flexion of the knees and hips (Figure 3.16). Unilateral flexion raise the suspicion of hip dysphasia or hemiparesis, whereas scissoring suggests spasticity.

CRANIAL NERVES

This is an important examination in newborns and babies, and is often overlooked. In particular, when using cranial adjusting, great changes in aberrant cranial nerve function can be observed. Part of the examination can be completed without touching the child, by simple observation and a history.

Cranial nerve I

Cranial nerve I is not normally assessed in infants.

Cranial nerve II

The eyes' response to light is assessed by the blink response. Fundoscopic examination is best carried out with the baby looking over the parent's shoulder; the examiner can then hold the head gently and examine the fundus.

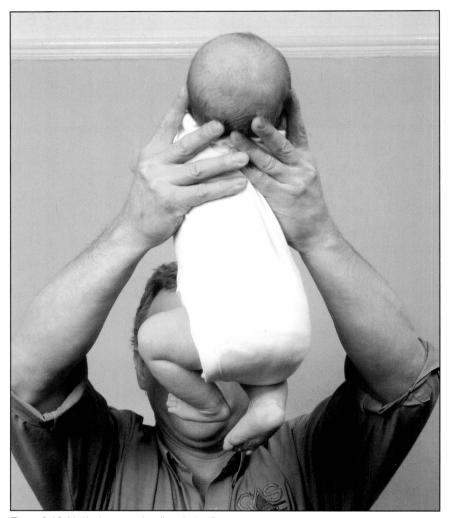

Figure 3.16 Vertical suspension (Landau) reflex.

Cranial nerves III, IV and VI

After the neonatal period, eye movements can be tested by moving an object from side to side and up and down about 45 cm (18 inches) from the baby's face. I use a brightly coloured abacus for this procedure. A neonate's eye movement can be tested using the dolls eye reflex in which movement of the head results in a deviation of the eyes in the opposite direction.

Eye problems including poor tracking and strabismus, and some types of nystagmus can occur after trauma to the sphenoid bone. Early cranial intervention is indicated.

Cranial nerves V, VII, IX, X and XII

The correct function of these nerves is demonstrated by healthy rooting, sucking, swallowing and gag reflexes. The corneal reflex involving cranial nerves V and VII can be demonstrated by gently blowing into one of

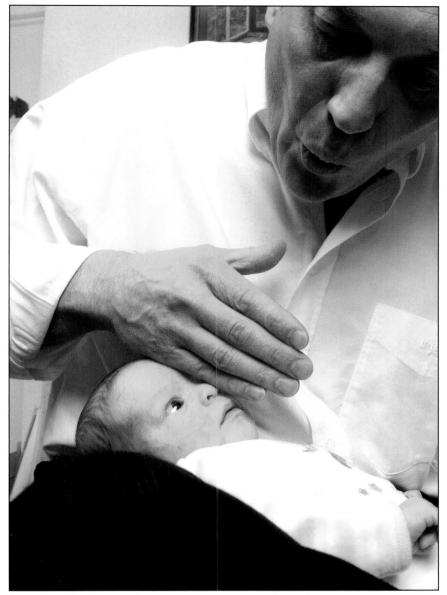

Figure 3.17 The Corneal reflex test.

the baby's eyes while shielding the other with your hand: both should blink (Figure 3.17).

Compression of the jugular foramen and the hypoglossal canal is a common lesion seen in infants and produces such symptoms as an inability to suck, gagging, poor swallowing and regurgitation. These often respond readily to cranial correction.

Cranial nerve VIII is difficult to assess accurately, but some indication of function is given by the acoustic blink reflex. An otoscopic examination should be performed in an infant who is distressed and pulls at its ear lobes. Glue ear is a very common finding in babies and young children; this results from a buckling of the temporal bone, which causes drainage

via the eustachian tube to be compromised. Both temporal decompression and upper cervical adjustment often prove helpful.

Functioning of cranial nerve XI is demonstrated by the infant's head posture and spontaneous activity. A head tilt and drooping of the shoulder are suggestive of lesions of the nerve. Jugular foramen compression and direct trauma to the sternocleidomastoid muscle are relatively common sequelae to a traumatic birth, producing a torticollis. These respond readily to early cranial intervention.

ORTHOPAEDIC TESTS

The two most important tests when examining neonates are Barlow's test and Ortolani's test, which both evaluate hip stability. These tests should not be performed repetitively for fear of increasing the hip instability and are mainly indicated for use in the neonatal period. In my experience, when hip instability is present, there will often be asymmetry of the fat creases in the baby's buttocks and anterior/posterior thigh. Severe sacral torsions can also cause these asymmetries.

Barlow's test

This tests for a hip that is unstable and able to dislocate. The test is performed with the infant supine and the hip adducted to the midline and flexed to 90 degrees (Figure 3.18). Pressure is directed posteriorly from the infant's knee into the table with two fingers at the posterior aspect of the hip joint to palpate for laxity or a click. If excessive laxity or a click is present, the hip is most likely to be unstable.

Ortolani's test

Ortolani's test tests whether the hip is dislocated. It is performed supine with the hip flexed to 90 degrees and fully abducted. Two fingers contact the posterior aspect of the infant's hip joint, and pressure is then gently applied from posterior to anterior to test for excessive laxity or a reduction click while the ligamentous barrier is gently stressed in full abduction. In my opinion, this test is better performed on one side at a time (Figure 3.19a), but it is often recommended that both hips should be examined at the same time (Figure 3.19b). In order to access the ligamentous end-feel, it is important that time is taken to allow the baby's muscular resistance to abate.

Carreiro (2003) notes that the hip joint has a 'rotator cuff' similar to that of the shoulder. The gluteus medius and minimus, attaching anteriorly to the femoral tubercle, act as abductors and internal rotators of the femur and stabilise the non-weight-bearing side of the pelvis during gait. The piriformis, gamelli, obturators and quadratus femoris attach to the posterior femur and act as external rotators. Together, they stabilise and guide the movement and position of the femoral head within the acetabulum. Abnormal tension or

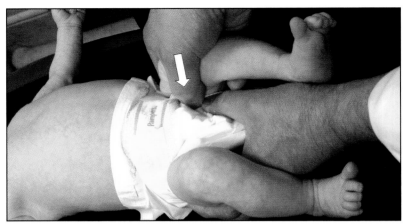
Figure 3.18 Barlow's test.

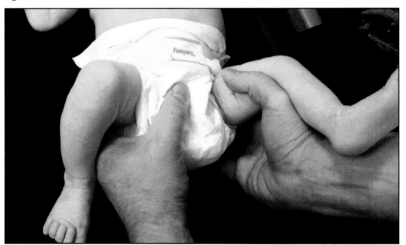
Figure 3.19a Ortolani's test: unilateral.

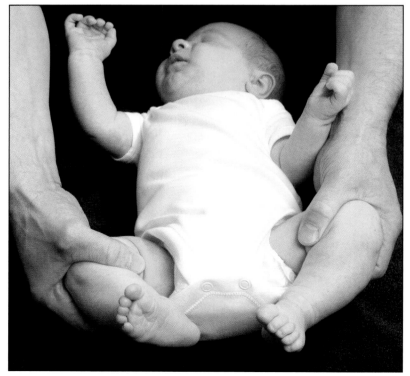
Figure 3.19b Ortolani's test: bilateral.

tone within these muscles will affect femoral stability within the acetabulum, so their function needs to be borne in mind when evaluating hip clicks in neonates.

Although referral is always indicated for a suspected unstable hip, this does not mean that treatment of the component parts of the innominate bone (pubis, ilia and ischia) and correction of the relevant hip musculature is not indicated. Many hip clicks stabilise with intervention, but referral for ultrasound or X-ray studies is still indicated.

SPINAL AND CRANIAL EXAMINATION

Both spinal and cranial examination will be covered in depth in Chapters 5 and 6.

REFERENCES

Anrig CA, Plaugher G (eds). *Pediatric Chiropractic*. Baltimore: Williams & Wilkins, 1998.

Ballard JL, Novak KK, Driver M. A simplified score of assessment of fetal maturation of newly born infants. *J Pediatr* 1979; 95: 769.

Carreiro JE. *An Osteopathic Approach to Children*. Edinburgh: Churchill Livingstone, 2003.

Goddard S. *Reflexes, Learning and Behaviour: A Window into a Child's Mind*. Eugene, Oregon: Fern Ridge Press, 2002.

Mocsary P, Gaal J, Komaroy B. Relationship between fetal intracranial pressure and fetal heart rate during labor. *Am J Obstet Gynecol* 1970; 106: 407–411.

Shumway-Cook A, Woollacott MH. *Motor Control: Theory and Practical Applications, 2nd edn*. New York: Lippincott Williams & Wilkins, 2000.

Illustrations in Chapter Three

Chapter 4
Common infant and neonatal signs and symptoms

Parents bring babies and children to chiropractic clinics for a wide variety of reasons, ranging from check-ups to serious health issues. In the UK, there has been much favourable publicity about chiropractic care for infant colic; this has led many health visitors and midwives to refer mothers to chiropractors so that their infants can be assessed and treated for colic and other related conditions. This, however, covers only a small percentage of the paediatric cases seen by chiropractors, and it is important that chiropractors are aware of commonly presenting symptomatology, where the potential areas of subluxation or lesion may be located and which tissues may be involved. This chapter will focus on the symptomatology of neonates and infants.

USING THE HISTORY

Details of the natal, neonatal and infant history given by the parent(s) provide the clinician with many clues on where to look therapeutically at the infant. The following should be regarded only as guidelines and do not substitute for a thorough examination and clinical impression. They do, however, act as good pointers as to what to look for.

- The infant suckles from one breast well but not the other. This is a common presentation in infants with rotary or lateral atlas subluxations. The mother will often be able to suckle the baby on the more difficult breast only by having it supported by the side of her on a cushion, so that the baby lies on the same side as when feeding from the other breast.

- The infant holds his or her head in lateral flexion or extension. This is again typical of an atlas subluxation and is a feature of KISS syndrome (see below).

- The infant dislikes lying supine. In my experience, this indicates a compression of the occiput. These babies tend to be very fussy and get upset when their head is touched or stroked, often objecting when a hat is put on them.

- The infant exhibits a poor sleep pattern and regularly wakes screaming. It is abnormal for babies to wake screaming as if they are having a nightmare; in the past, this has been referred to as the child having night terrors. In my experience, the primary lesion is occipital compression.

- The infant suckles only briefly and the mouth does not cover much of the areola of the nipple. This is typical of a temporomandibular joint problem. It is important because the infant will only receive the foremilk and not the more nutritive hindmilk. The baby will tend to show a mandibular deviation on full opening.

- The infant exhibits a weak suck. This is a common problem, typical of an occipital condylar compression (Magoun 1976, Arbuckle 1994, Frymann 1998). The condylar canal carrying the hypoglossal nerve is generally involved.

- The infant exhibits an excessively strong suck. The classic symptom in these cases is the mother's complaints of abnormally sore and often cracked nipples (be sure that the mother does not have a fungal infection of the nipple such as candidiasis, which is quite common). This is usually the result of a compression of the infant's maxillae. The mother is very grateful when the problem is sorted out!

- The infant coughs and chokes while feeding. This is a sign of jugular foramen compression (Arbuckle 1994), usually as a result of disruption of the component parts of the occiput irritating the glossopharyngeal and possibly the vagus nerve.

- Infant colic. This is generally caused by compression of the jugular foramen, as above, leading to vagal irritation. Upper cervical involvement is common.

- Repetitive vomiting after feeding. According to Frymann (1998), this is a sign of occipital condylar compression influencing the vagus nerve. Soft tissue involvement, especially excessive tightness at the respiratory diaphragm, is also a regular finding.

- Hypertonia (a nervous, crying, sleepless, tense baby). The pyramidal tracts lie in close proximity to the basilar portion of the occiput. Frymann (1998) postulates that hypertonia is caused when occipital condylar compression influences these tracts. In my experience, infants who startle easily, especially those who have a hyperactive Moro response, will commonly show severe torsion of the sphenoid bone.

- Hypotonia (floppy baby syndrome). The extrapyramidal tracts are situated laterally in the medulla oblongata. Frymann (1998, p 101) states that 'hypotonia may be the earliest manifestation of their dysfunction' and relates this dysfunction to occipital condylar compression.

- The infant is distressed on having the nappy (diaper) changed. This is a classic sign of a sacral subluxation in infants. They object to having their hips flexed and their legs abducted.

- Constipation/diarrhoea. This can be from sacral or thoraco-lumbar subluxations, or jugular foramen compression (occipital condylar compression).

- Glue ear. Glue ear commonly involves lesions of the temporal bone and the cranial base (Carreiro 2003). Upper cervical involvement, especially of C2, is also common.

- Strabismus. This often involves lesions of the sphenoid bone, although any of the bones surrounding the orbit can be involved.

KISS SYNDROME

German medical doctors who are practitioners of manual medicine have written some of the most interesting and persuasive research utilising the chiropractic technique. Biedermann (1992) coined the phrase 'kinematic imbalances due to suboccipital strain' (KISS) syndrome when referring to a wide variety of symptoms suffered by infants that appear to have their origin in the upper cervical spine.

Symptoms of KISS are:

- head tilt/torticollis;
- opisthotonos – the head is held in extension and the baby is unable to lie on his or her back;
- a uniform sleeping position, the child crying if the mother tries to change its position;
- asymmetrical motor patterns;
- an asymmetrical posture of the trunk and extremities;

- sleeping disorders: the baby regularly wakes crying through the night;

- extreme sensitivity of the neck;

- cranial scoliosis;

- blockages (fixations) of the sacroiliac joints and asymmetries of the gluteal muscles;

- an asymmetrical development and range of motion of the hip joints;

- fever of unknown origin and loss of appetite.

Beidermann (1992) qualifies this by stating that these symptoms cover a wide range of pathological conditions and cannot always be attributable to the upper cervical spine, but when encountered in a combination of motor asymmetries, sleep disorders and cranial asymmetry, it is worthwhile looking at the upper cervical spine.

Beidermann (2005) has more recently refined and subdivided KISS syndrome into KISS 1 and KISS 2, reflecting the different parameters he has observed.

In KISS 1, the major marker exhibited is fixed lateral flexion/rotation of the head. This may be accompanied by unilateral microsomia, asymmetry of the skull, scoliosis of the neck and trunk, gluteal area asymmetry, asymmetrical limb movements and a retardation of motor development on one side.

The major marker shown by children with KISS 2 is fixed cervical hyperextension during sleep. This may be accompanied by asymmetrical occipital flattening, pulled-up shoulders, fixed supination of the arms, difficulty in lifting the trunk when prone, orofacial muscle hypotonia and difficulty breast-feeding from one side.

The KISS syndromes demonstrate how far-reaching the effects of upper cervical subluxations can be. They are, however, limited to the upper cervical complex, and if we include the effects of occipital, temporal, sphenoid and other cranial lesions, we get much further in evaluating the health status of the infant or child. I believe we see every day in our practices the consequences of not correcting individuals as babies, older children and adults presenting with a myriad of preventable back pain, headaches, digestive problems, learning and behavioural disorders and other impediments to their quality of life.

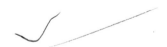

REFERENCES

Arbuckle BE. *The Selected Writings of Beryl E Arbuckle*. Indianapolis: American Academy of Osteopathy, 1994.

Biedermann H. Kinematic imbalances due to suboccipital strain in newborns. *Manipulative Med* 1992; 6: 151–156.

Biedermann H. Manual therapy in children: proposals for an etiologic model. *J Manipulative Physiol Ther* 2005; 28: e1–e15.

Carreiro JE. *An Osteopathic Approach to Children*. Edinburgh: Churchill Livingstone, 2003.

Frymann V. *The Collected Writings of Viola M Frymann*. Indianapolis: American Academy of Osteopathy, 1998.

Magoun HI. *Osteopathy in the Cranial Field*. Indianapolis: Cranial Academy, 1976.

Chapter 5
Spinal examination and correction

When examining a newborn infant (up to 3 weeks of age), one of the most important procedures is observation. Lie the infant on your adjusting table or on the floor and observe him or her. Babies will often take on the distortion pattern that they held in utero (due to constraint), and you can observe which regions have fascial restrictions that need attention (Philips 1999).

INVERTED HANG

The inverted hang (DeJarnette 1979) is a test that is used extensively in the chiropractic profession and can give some very useful results, but it needs to be used with caution. It is absolutely contraindicated in haemorrhagic disease of the newborn or any other condition involving bleeding or haemorrhage. Inversion should also be avoided if there is hydrocephalus, hip instability or neurological symptoms, for example epilepsy. That said, the test provides, in not too severely compromised babies, definitive indications of where a lesion is located and where to focus treatment.

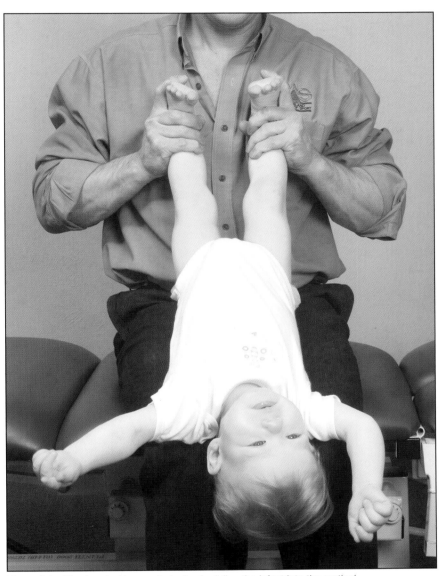

Figure 5.1a The inverted hang: start, slowly sliding the infant into the vertical.

Method

The baby should lie supine on the chiropractic doctor's lap, with the soles of the feet facing the doctor's body. The lower limbs (not just the ankles) are gripped so that the feet can be dorsiflexed (using a pistol grip with the forefinger performing the dorsiflexion). The doctor, sitting on the edge of the bench, gradually drops his or her knees lower so that the baby angles down towards the floor without being startled (Figure 5.1a). Slowly, the doctor lifts the baby up by the legs so that he or she hangs in inversion over the doctor's lap (if the baby is small enough) or over the bench or floor (Figure 5.1b). The baby is then gently returned to the doctor's lap, the doctor's knees being used as the fulcrum to lie the head back down. This can be a little tricky if the infant goes into hyperextension so the parent may need to guide and support the infant's head.

The doctor should explain the procedure and reassure the parents (particularly first-time parents) prior to performing the inversion: I will never forget having a mother burst into tears when she saw her beloved baby inverted.

Results

- The head rotates in one direction: subluxation of C1–C2 (change the baby's position first to make sure that he or she is not looking at Mum).
- The head is held in lateral flexion: occipital condyle or cervical facet subluxation (kinematic imbalances due to suboccipital strain (KISS I).
- The neck is in extension: occipital condylar compression (KISS II).
- The neck is held in flexion: cranial dural restriction.
- The baby's trunk adopts a laterally flexed or twisted posture: thoracic/rib subluxation and/or body fascial restriction.
- The leg lengths are uneven: pelvic ligamentous injury/instability.

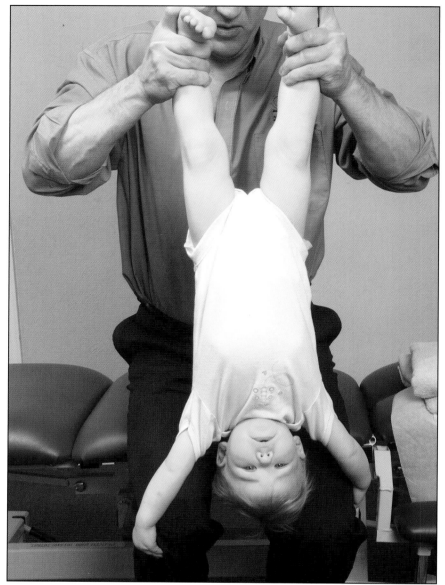

Figure 5.1b The inverted hang: finishing position.

Most babies, certainly those below 6 months of age, should 'enjoy' being hung upside down; if this distresses them, this is another sign of a cranial restriction or compression.

As long as the baby tolerates the procedure well, the inverted hang can be shown to parents as home therapy. It tractions out minor spinal and pelvic restrictions and increases blood and cerebrospinal fluid flow into the cranium, which raises the intracranial pressure and can be used to help minor cranial restrictions. The parents should be instructed to invert the baby (over a bed for safety, and with another person present) and swing him or her gently backwards and forwards for 15 seconds. The procedure is then repeated and can be performed every day.

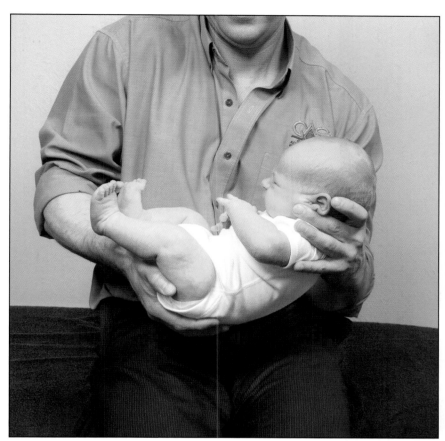

Figure 5.2 Testing infant trunk flexion.

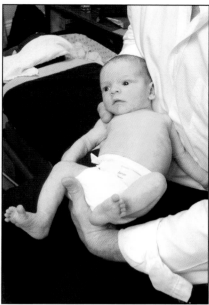

Figure 5.3 Testing right lateral trunk flexion.

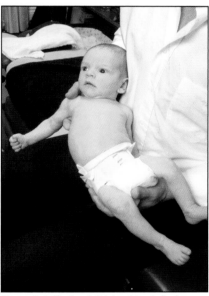

Figure 5.4 Testing left lateral trunk flexion.

ASSESSMENT OF TRUNK FLEXIBILITY

This procedure (which can be used up to 3 months of age) is a very useful method of finding and correcting fascial restrictions occasioned by intrauterine constraint.

Method

The baby is held by the doctor, one hand under the pelvis and the other hand under the shoulders, neck and occiput. The baby is gently flexed and extended, ease of motion and restriction being ascertained (Figure 5.2). The baby is then laterally flexed at the trunk to the left and right (Figures 5.3 and 5.4), the trunk next being twisted to the left and right. Restriction in any direction is noted.

Correction

If, for example, the baby is restricted in left lateral flexion, the baby is taken gently into right flexion (the direction of freedom) as far as possible until a release is felt in that direction. If the baby begins 'unwinding', follow this until the unwinding stops. The unwinding follows the pattern of restriction of the infant's fascia as it releases; it can lead to some bizarre movement patterns on the part of the infant, but if it occurs it is important to follow the infant's movement until the unwinding stops and the infant relaxes. The infant will sometimes become distressed while unwinding so reassure the parents that the infant is fine. The restriction in left lateral flexion should now be free.

This principle is applied to all directions of restriction: go into the opposite free direction until it releases or unwinds and then re check the areas of previous restriction.

THE CERVICAL SPINE

Assessment

In older children who can sit still, conventional static and motion palpation procedures can be employed, but in infants this is not the case. With younger babies, the easiest method is for the doctor to cross one leg over, ankle on to thigh, in a figure 4 and sit the baby in the recess formed. The baby's head is held over the fronto-parietal area, while the other hand presses the infant's transverse processes individually from T1 to C1, posterior to anterior, feeling for pliability. Any rotation, bilateral subluxation or restriction is then easily palpated (Figure 5.5).

Treatment

On the cervical spines of young infants, I tend to use adjustments without auditory osseous releases as these can be scary for parents who may not be patients themselves. They often imagine that this will hurt or damage the baby, although we know that this is not the case. Low-force adjusting techniques are also, in the main, more effective on infants and do not distress them.

This type of low-force cervical adjusting is a direct method using both slow-stretch and fast-stretch

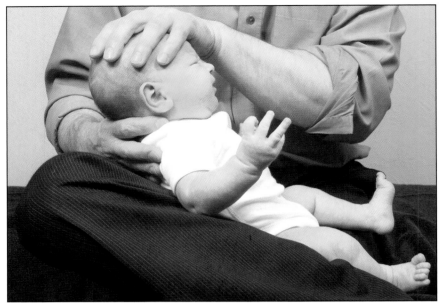

Figure 5.5 Cervical spine palpation in an infant.

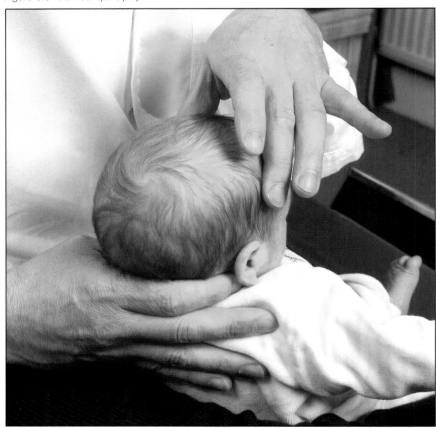

Figure 5.6 Cervical spine correction in an infant.

techniques, the correction taking place in the same position as for cervical palpation. The side of restriction is identified, and gentle pressure is used into that restriction. After a few seconds, a soft tissue 'give' is felt; this is then 'set' with a fast-stretch flick in the same direction (Figure 5.6).

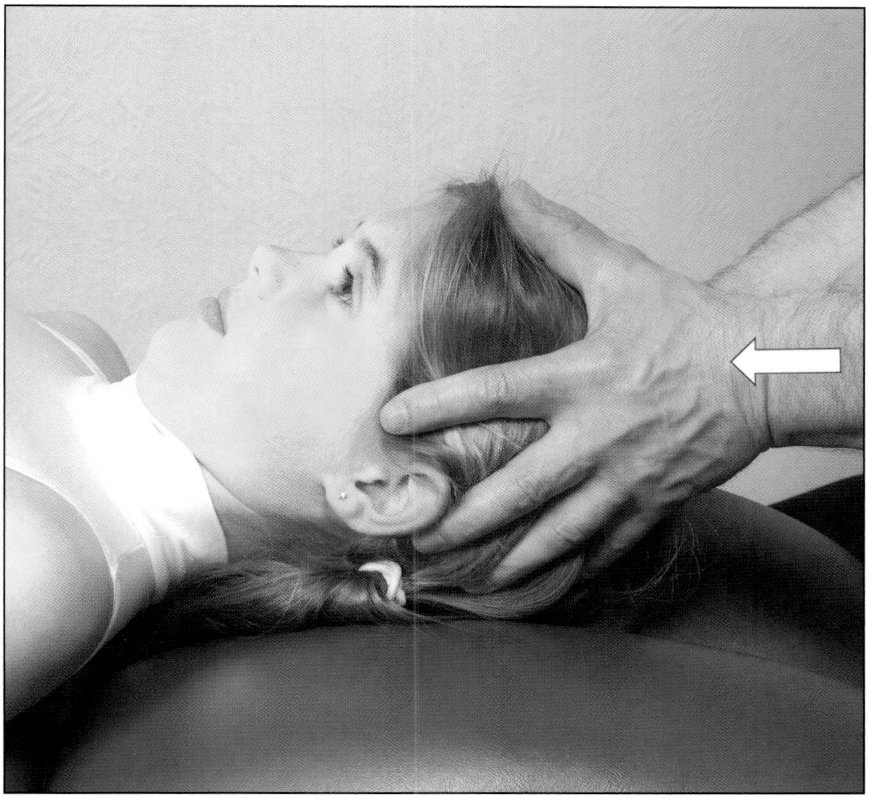

The cervical stair-step (De-Jarnette 1984) can be used for children 2 or more years of age and is an excellent method for assessing and correcting the cervical spine in older children. The child lies supine, and the doctor takes whole-hand contacts over the parietal bones, with the fingers spread either side of the child's ears. Pressure is then directed caudally towards the child's feet (Figure 5.7). The child's head should rise in four distinct steps towards the ceiling:

- Step 1 C7-T1.
- Step 2 C5-C6.
- Step 3 C3-C4.
- Step 4 C1-C2.

Progression should be smooth and steady, with no 'jumps' or restrictions.

C0–C1 can be assessed as well by extending the occiput on the cervical spine at the end of the other four steps.

Any levels of restriction noted, or a jump causing a missed step, should be addressed. The stair-step movement is held just prior to the jump or restriction, and a figure-of-8 movement involving lateral flexion and rotation is employed. This should free up the restriction and allow a gentle glide through all four steps.

THORACIC SPINE

Both motion and static palpation of the thoracic and lumbar spine in infants can be problematic; we

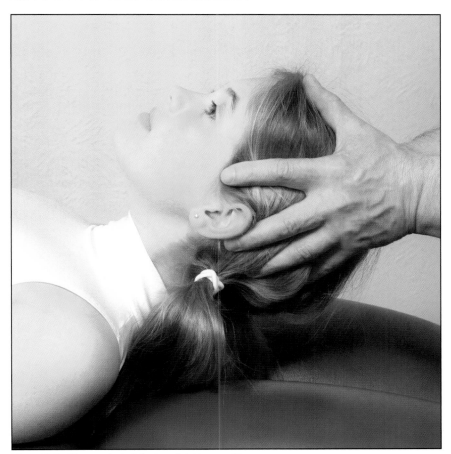

Figure 5.7a The cervical stair-step: starting position.

Figure 5.7b The cervical stair-step: finishing position.

therefore need to apply special techniques for this.

Assessment

The easiest method of palpating the ribs and thoracic and lumbar spine in an infant is with the lying baby prone over the doctor's lap. The infant's head and face hang over the lateral edge of one thigh, facing the floor (Figure 5.8). The doctor's legs are then slowly opened and closed by a few centimetres; this creates some extension in the spine and ribs and allows motion and any restrictions present to be assessed. This is useful as far up the spine as T1 and as low as L5.

This is also a good position to perform static palpation and assess any static rotations or malpositions.

Treatment

The thoracic spine at T3–L1 is most easily adjusted using the weight of the infant to assist with the correction. The doctor gently extends the infant over his or her hip or thigh; this allows tension to be introduced into the involved segment. The areas of subluxation – spine or ribs – are contacted with two fingers on either side (rotation can be corrected by primarily contacting only one side). A supination flick of the wrists performs the adjustment, usually with an audible osseous release (Figure 5.9a).

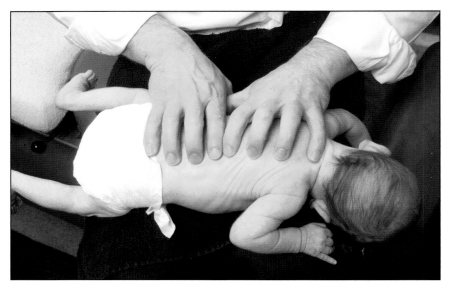

Figure 5.8 Lumbo-thoracic palpation.

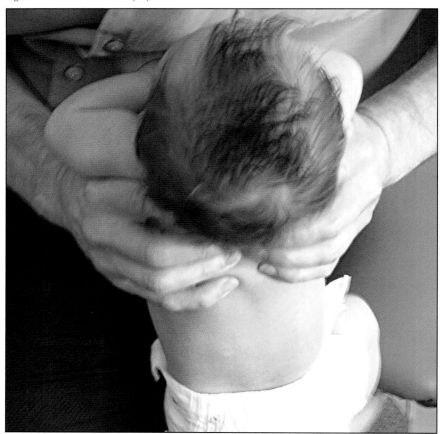

Figure 5.9a Thoracic adjustment – neonate.

With slightly older infants who need less stabilisation and have more body weight, the doctor can just lift the infant up in front of him or her and adjust the involved vertebral level with the supination wrist-flick. This can also be performed with the baby facing away from the doctor, who then uses the thumbs to contact the involved vertebra (Figure 5.9b). A wrist pronation flick is then used to complete the adjustment.

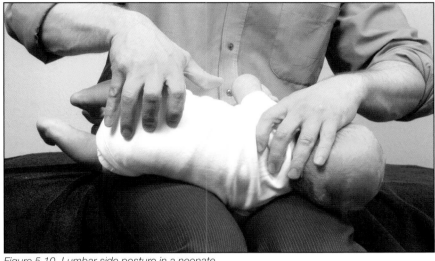

Figure 5.10 Lumbar side posture in a neonate.

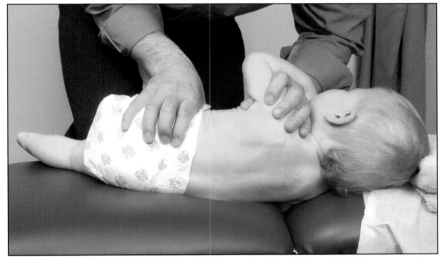

Figure 5.11 Lumbar side posture in an infant or toddler.

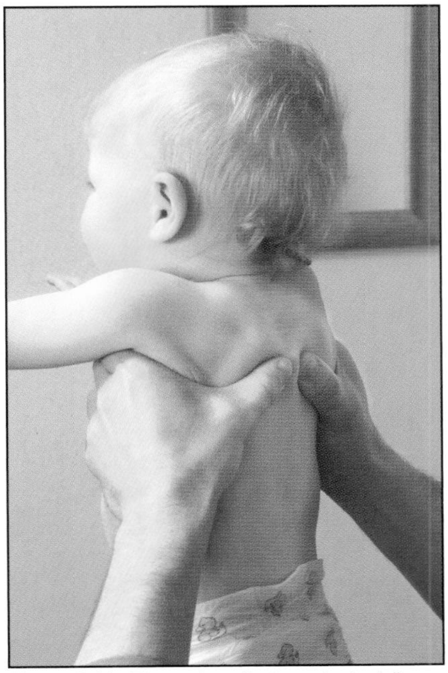

LUMBAR SPINE

Palpation of the lumbar spine is performed in infants as described previously for the thoracic spine.

Treatment

Rotational subluxation of the lumbar spine (and sacrum) is easily addressed in young infants in a side-posture position. This is accomplished with small infants side-lying in the doctor's lap (Figure 5.10) on the side of spinous rotation or anterior sacrum, with the baby's inferior arm stabilised and held between the doctor's thighs. The upper shoulder is held with one hand, the infant's upper leg being flexed and the pelvis stabilised with the doctor's wrist. Contact is made with the posterior mamillary process or sacrum using the first two fingers of the doctor's inferior hand. Tension is taken up and a gentle 'flick' adjustment is given, usually with an audible osseous release.

Older infants are better adjusted on an adjusting table. Again, the infant's flexed leg is stabilised by the doctor's hand, rather than using the doctor's leg, as would be done when adjusting adults (Figure 5.11).

If an osseous adjustment is not indicated, lumbar subluxations can be corrected by holding the involved spinous process in the direction of correction until a soft tissue release is felt; this can be followed up by a fast-stretch flick.

Figure 5.9b Thoracic adjustment – toddler.

REFERENCES

DeJarnette MB. *Cranial Technique*. Private publication, Nebraska City, USA, 1979.

Dejarnette MB. *Sacro Occipital Technique*. Private publication, Nebraska City, USA, 1984.

Phillips CE. *Paediatrics lecture*, Anglo-European College of Chiropractic, Bournemouth,1999.

Illustrations in Chapter Five

Figure 5.1	The inverted hang: (a) starting and (b) finishing positions.
Figure 5.2	Testing infant trunk flexion.
Figure 5.3	Testing right lateral trunk flexion.
Figure 5.4	Testing left lateral trunk flexion.
Figure 5.5	Cervical spine palpation in an infant.
Figure 5.6	Cervical spine correction in an infant.
Figure 5.7	The cervical stair-step: (a) starting and (b) finishing positions.
Figure 5.8	Lumbo-thoracic palpation.
Figure 5.9a	Thoracic adjustment- neonate
Figure 5.9b	Thoracic adjustment- toddler.
Figure 5.10	Lumbar side posture in a neonate.
Figure 5.11	Lumbar side posture in an infant or toddler.

Chapter 6
Examination and correction of the craniosacral system

THE BASICS

Many chiropractors feel discouraged from undertaking cranial work as they feel it takes too long to master the subtleties of palpating cranial motion. Nothing, however, is further from the truth – although it might take a lifetime to master all aspects of cranial work, the basics of treating babies and children can be gained in a fairly short time by having an open mind and a little application.

Many organisations offer detailed training courses in cranial work, and these are certainly well worth undertaking, but I am convinced that most chiropractors can easily master two or three basic cranial decompressions, which will allow them to correct many of the complaints of the paediatric patient. The ability to palpate the cranial rhythmic impulse (CRI) is not a prerequisite to the successful cranial adjusting of infants and children. This can in fact be exceedingly difficult; indeed, I was not convinced of my own ability to palpate the CRI in babies for my first 8 years in

cranial paediatrics, but I still had success. The most critical aspect is the ability to palpate tissue tension and unwind the restriction, literally following the tissue into the direction of 'freedom', as will be seen later in this chapter.

THE CRANIAL RHYTHMIC IMPULSE

Cranial work in the modern era dates back to the 1930s when William G. Sutherland D.O. and Nephri Cottam D.C. both published on the subject of cranial correction (Pederick 1997). Cranial bone motion and the CRI have been demonstrated in many human and animal studies (Tettambel et al 1978, Lewer Allen and Bunt 1979, Podlas et al 1984, Adams et al 1992, Heisey and Adams 1993, Lewandowski et al 1996). The CRI is a wave-like pulsation through the craniosacral system not synchronous with cardiovascular or respiratory motion. It is usually quoted as being between 4 and 16 cycles per minute (Chaitow 1999).

The question of how the CRI is actually generated has produced many theories:

- Sutherland (1939) believed that involuntary brain motion generated a pulse wave of cerebrospinal fluid (CSF), which caused motion within the dural membrane system and subsequently in the cranium and sacrum. Motion of the cranium was dependent on mobility at the cranial sutures and the patency of the reciprocal tension membranes of the skull.

- Lumsden (1951) postulated that the CRI was generated by oligodendrite cell coiling/uncoiling. These oligodendrite cells certainly do appear to possess an inherent motion, but this motion would seem to be too little to be solely responsible for the generation of the CRI.

- Magoun (1976) proposed that an electrical current or magnetic field produced the brain motion that Sutherland espoused. He also believed that variations in the production of CSF in the choroid plexus influenced brain mobility and the CRI.

- Upledger (Upledger and Vredevoogd 1983), widely known for his writings and teachings in the realm of craniosacral therapy, used aspects of Magoun's CSF production variation theory and formulated the pressurestat hypothesis, in which variations in the production and absorption of CSF drive the rhythmic brain motion. This theory is one of the most widely accepted theories of CRI generation, but some doubts have been raised over whether the amount of CSF produced is enough by itself to drive the CRI (Feinberg and Mark 1987).

- Ferguson (1991) suggested that there was a muscular origin to the CRI. It is easy to understand how there may, on active movement, be a muscular component to the CRI; this does not, however, explain how we are able to palpate the CRI in cases of quadriplegia and coma.

- Degenhardt and Kuchera (1996) noted that there was an inherent contractility within the lymphatic system and that this might be the origin of the CRI. This again, however, may be too small an impulse on its own to produce the CRI.

- McPartland and Mein (1997) describe a theory of CRI generation known as the entrainment hypothesis. This is one of the most recent additions to the vexed question of what produces the CRI and may well prove to be the most complete. It is in some ways a conglomeration of previous theories rather than an alter-

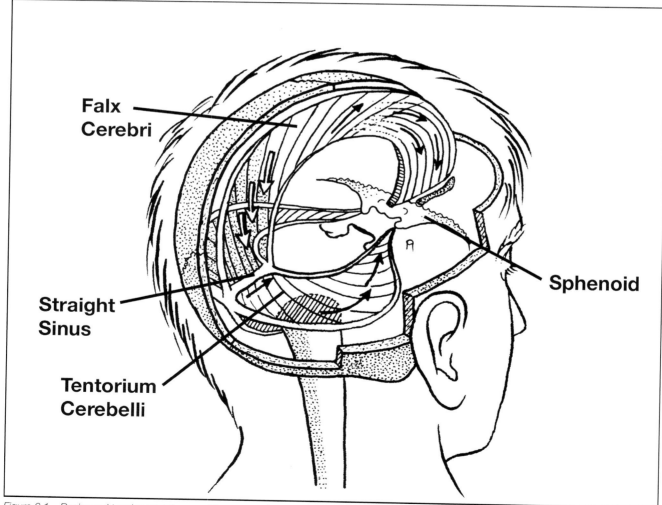

Figure 6.1   Reciprocal tension membranes. The arrows show the lines of force that may act on these during flexion. Adapted from Gehin: Atlas of Manipulative Techniques for the Cranium and Face.

native view. McPartland and Mein's hypothesis is that CRI is the product of multiple biological rhythms or oscillators, producing the entrainment, or integration and harmonisation, of these oscillators. The biological oscillators include cortical oxidative metabolism, respiration, cardiovascular motion, lymphatic motion, muscular contraction and the electromagnetic field interaction between doctor and patient. The primary mechanism responsible for the generation of these biological oscillators is the balance between the sympathetic and parasympathetic nervous systems. It is interesting that this balance is suggested to be the primary driving force as it may explain the wide variations in CRI rate and amplitude.

Cranial Motion

When discussing the CRI and cranial motion, we are talking about not simply interbone motion at the sutures, but also the movement of the reciprocal tension membranes within the cranium itself (Figure 6.1). This is particularly important when dealing with infants, in whom there is as yet no sutural interdigitation. These membranes are under continuous dynamic tension so a change in one requires an adaptive change in the others. In flexion (the inhalation phase), the tentorium

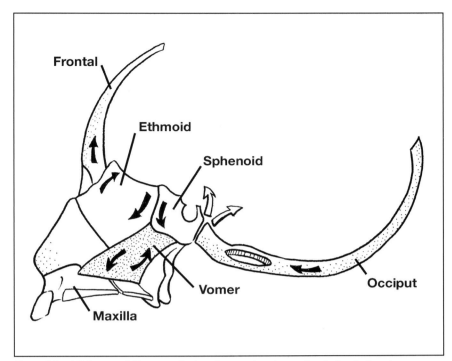

Figure 6.2   Midline cranial bones – flexion. Arrows showing motion in the flexion phase. Adapted from Gehin: Atlas of Manipulative Techniques for the Cranium and Face.

cerebelli flattens and the falx cerebri shortens from front to back, the process then reversing in extension (the exhalation phase).

Flexion within the cranium occurs when the sphenobasilar symphysis elevates, with the occiput and sphenoid bone rotating in opposite directions. During flexion, the greater wings of the sphenoid move in an anterior–inferior direction, with the sphenoid body moving superior, as the sphenobasilar symphysis rises. The basilar portion of the occiput rises in flexion, and intrabone flexion occurs as the squama approximates the basilar portion. It is controversial whether this occurs in the same way after the age of 25 years, when the symphysis is fully ossified

(Chaitow 1999), but that is not a concern in terms of paediatrics. The ethmoid rotates in the direction opposite to that of the sphenoid, causing the vomer to come under tension.

The actual rotational motion of the vomer (important for our inter oral cranial adjustments) appears to be of some debate. Magoun (1976) and Chaitow (1999) show the posterior edge of the vomer moving inferiorly in flexion, whereas Gehin (1985) and Howat (1999) show it moving in a superior direction. After looking carefully at the anatomy and experimenting with skull corrections, it seems that the latter theory is most likely to be correct (Figure 6.2).

The paired bones (including the temporals, parietals, zygoma and maxillae) generally rotate away from the midline in flexion. The temporal squama slides postero-inferiorly, and the mastoid tips approximate and move anteriorly in flexion, with the process reversed in extension.

The motion of the parietal bones is somewhat reminiscent of the movement of a bird's wing, with their inferior edges moving apart and superiorly in flexion about an axis of the sagittal suture. The maxillae have a motion similar to that of the parietals about the axis of the intermaxillary suture, but their motion is complicated by their articulation with the vomer. In flexion, the anterior parts of the maxillae move inferiorly, with the posterior parts moving superiorly.

CRANIAL EXAMINATION

Particularly in young infants, the cranium should be observed for symmetry, initially from above. The nose should be in line with the fontanelles; the ears should be in line with each other and reasonably flat to the head. The overall shape of the head should be oval, and any deviations from this should be noted as they can indicate where the cranial strain originates.

When analysed from the front, the skull should be looked at for the levels of the ears, eyes and maxillae. The easiest way to do this is for the doctor to put his or her fingers in the baby's ears and level the head; with the thumb tips placed on the lateral frontal notches, any distortion in the skull's rear pivot (the

sphenobasilar symphysis) can be demonstrated by an uneven distance between the thumb and finger on either side.

The level of the maxilla is more difficult to ascertain in babies. Some guidance can be gained by observing the edge of baby's mouth when he or she cries or smiles: the higher side will tend to indicate the higher maxilla. Digital examination within the mouth can also prove useful. In an older child, putting a tongue compressor or pencil behind the canine (eye) teeth will give a good idea of maxillary level.

The relative levels of the maxillae and eyes (sphenoid bone) tell us what is going on in the anterior pivot of the skull (sphenomaxillary junction).

Skull pivots

The skull base has front and rear 'pivots' through which strain patterns in the horizontal and vertical planes occur (Figure 6.3). These are located at the sphenobasilar symphysis (rear pivot) and the sphenomaxillary junction (front pivot). This divides the skull into three sections: rear (occiput and temporal bones), middle (sphenoid and frontal bones) and anterior (maxillae and facial complex).

Neonatal skull

The neonatal skull is designed for passage through the birth canal, enabling it to mould in a quite amazing way and also to protect the brain, brainstem and cranial nerves. The skull base is

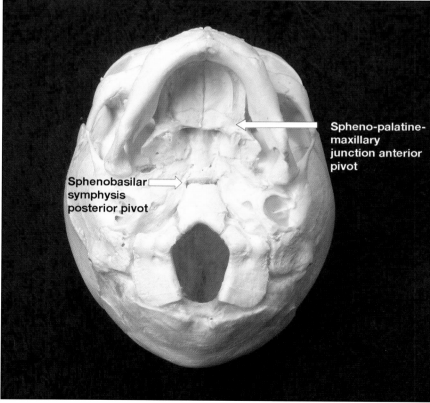

Figure 6.3 Anterior and posterior skull pivots.

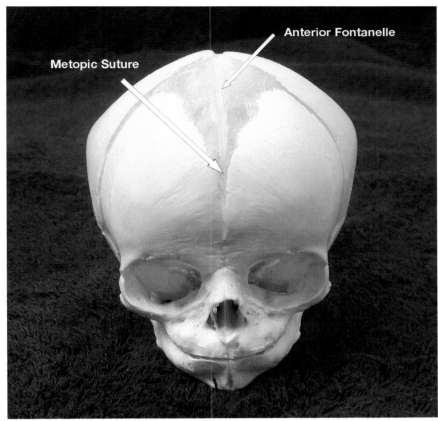

Figure 6.4 Superior view of a fetal skull, showing the anterior fontanelle.

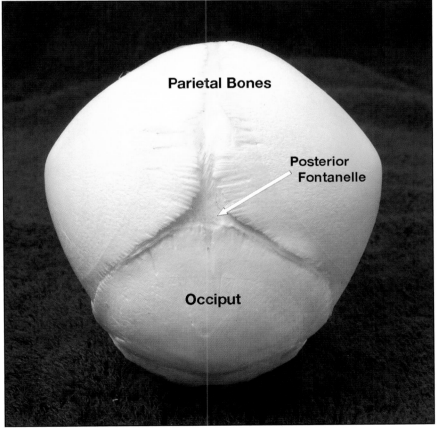

Figure 6.5 Posterior view of a fetal skull, showing the posterior fontanelle.

formed from cartilage and the neurocranium from membrane. This allows structural stability for the skull base, protecting the delicate nervous and vascular structures passing through the skull's foramina and allowing plasticity and pliability of the skull vault for passage down the birth canal.

The skull sutures do not interdigitate at this time (full interdigitation not being complete until about 7 years of age), and the cranial plates have fibrous tissue lying between them. There are a number of fontanelles or soft spots – the sphenoid fontanelle, mastoid fontanelle and anterior and posterior fontanelles – which allow the cranial plates to move and approximate during the birth process (Figures 6.4, 6.5 and 6.6). These fontanelles allow us to palpate the dura within the cranium to assess for raised intracranial pressure or dehydration. The neonatal skull vault provides a reflection of the dural system underneath. The vault bones adhere strongly to the dura and, because there is no interdigitation of sutures, respond to the stress patterns that the dura imposes.

The cartilaginous base of the cranium is made up of the occiput, petrous temporal and sphenoid bones. The occiput is in four parts: two condylar portions and one basilar portion formed from cartilage, and the squamous portion, formed mainly from membrane. The temporal bone has its petrous portions and tympanic ring formed from cartilage, and its squama formed from membrane. The sphenoid body and processes are cartilaginous in origin, but the greater wings originate in membrane.

The four occipital bones form a ring around the spinal cord at the foramen magnum and articulate with the atlas so they are both a fulcrum and a strain point. The occiput then forms junctions with the petrous temporal bone and the sphenoid body interspaced with fibrous tissue (Figure 6.7).

As the head descends during the birth process, the blood and CSF are progressively squeezed from the cranium. The spaces between the fontanelles narrow, and the frontal bones (a metopic suture creating two frontal bones at this stage) and occipital squama begin to 'telescope' under the parietal bones. It was previously thought that the parietal bones overlapped each other as well during the birth process, but research by Carlan et al (1991) shows that they abut tightly together to protect the brain. The suboccipito-bregmatic diameter shortens, and the mento-vertical diameter lengthens, because of the progressive intrabone flexion of the squamous occiput and frontal bones (Carlan et al 1991).

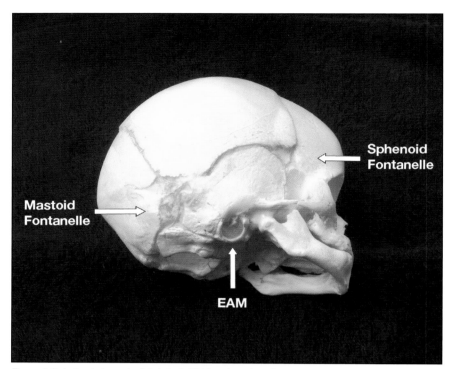

Figure 6.6 Lateral view of a fetal skull. EAM, external auditory meatus.

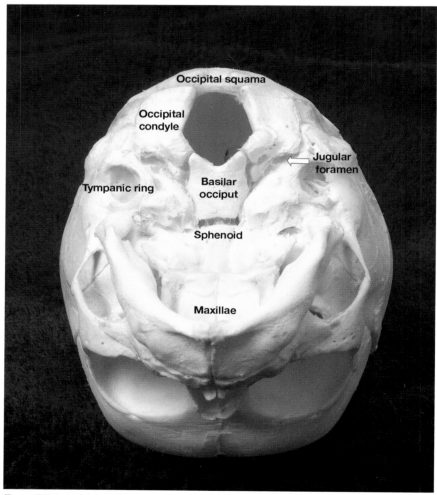

Figure 6.7 Late fetal skull base.

In summary, the skull lengthens from under the jaw to the back of the head, and shortens from the occiput to the top of the head.

The newborn's skull should regain symmetry within a few hours; any persistent asymmetry or persistent overriding after 24 hours is an indication for cranial therapeutic intervention (Upledger 1996).

If an infant becomes stuck with his or her head in an ascended or asynclistic position, this can create a strain on or distortion of the condylar portions of the occiput (Carriero 2003). A distortion of the occipital condyles can produce stress and compression of the jugular foramen or the hypoglossal canals (Magoun 1976, Arbuckle 1994, Carriero 2003). This condylar distortion will have an effect on the basilar portion and therefore have the potential, via the sphenobasilar symphysis, to create distortions of the sphenoid bone and the nerve supply to the eyes and their muscles, creating many of the eye problems we observe in infants and children.

SACRAL CORRECTION

The sacrum should be corrected before any cranial work proceeds as negative reactions to cranial work (usually minor ones) often occur because the sacrum has not been properly addressed. This is because of the sacrum's reciprocity with the occiput and its ability to create changes in cranial mechanics. It is therefore advisable to begin with sacral correction.

A classic sign of a severe sacral subluxation is that the mother complains that she is unable to change the baby's nappy (diaper) very easily. The baby often cries when its hips are flexed and its legs abducted in order to cleanse the anogenital area.

Examination

Remove or pull down the nappy, squeeze the buttocks together at mid-buttock level and observe the gluteal cleft (Figure 6.8): deviation of the cleft to either side indicates an anterior sacrum on that side. There is also often poor lower body flexibility and sometimes an unwillingness to abduct the knees with the hip and knees flexed. Asymmetrical fat creases may be apparent on the thighs or over the sacrum in the presence of hip pathology. This can also be caused by a lesion of the sacrum.

Sacral motion is assessed initially by placing the infant supine and testing each sacroiliac joint for pliability. One ilium is grasped over the posterior superior iliac spine by one of the doctor's hands, and the sacrum on that side is sheared against it using the other hand. This is repeated on the opposite side. The pliability of each joint is assessed, the restricted side being the one to be corrected.

Correction

If the sacrum is anterior on the restricted side, a contact is made with four fingers on the opposite or posterior side of the sacrum. The ileum on the anterior sacral side is then stabilised. Pressure is exerted on the posterior sacrum into correction (a direct technique) until a soft tissue release or 'give' is felt; this is reinforced with a wrist flexor flick with the

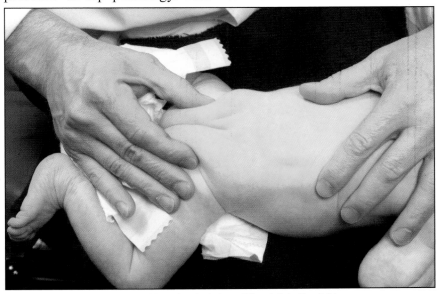

Figure 6.8 Sacral examination. Note the deviation of the cleft to the right.

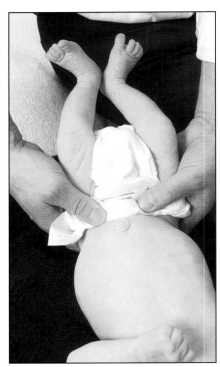

Figure 6.9 Sacral examination and correction.

sacral contact hand to 'set' the adjustment (Figure 6.9).

If the sacrum is posterior on the restricted side, the contact is with four fingers on the posterior sacrum side, the other hand stabilising the ipsilateral ileum. The rest of the adjustment proceeds as above.

Sacral segments

Examination

The sacral segments are not fused in babies and infants, and often need to be corrected individually after the adjustment of the sacrum as a whole. In my experience, S2 and S3 are the most frequently subluxated, possibly owing to their position at the apex of the sacral curve and the use of car seats. This can have significant effects for the

rest of the body because of the dural attachment at S2.

These segments are assessed by two single-finger contacts from each hand on either side of the sacral tubercles. One finger at a time pushes postero-anteriorly to assess pliability; any rotation or restriction of a segment is noted.

Correction

Correction of a sacral segment takes place with the hands in the same position as for the assessment. The side of posterior restriction is pressed anteriorly and held until a soft tissue 'give' is felt, when a fast-stretch 'flick' (via the wrist flexors) is given to set the adjustment. If the sacral segment as a whole is posterior, the postero-anterior pressure is

directed by both fingers on to both sides of the segment, and the adjustment is completed as above.

Sacral flexion and extension

This assesses the respiratory flexion–extension movement of the sacrum about an axis of the second sacral segment.

Assessment and correction

To open the posterior aspect of the sacroiliac joints and encourage flexion–extension, the doctor's hand contacts the supine infant's anterior superior iliac spines and squeezes them gently together. The doctor's other hand cups the sacrum (with a nappy in situ!); this hand gently flexes and extends the sacrum to encourage the motion (Figure 6.10).

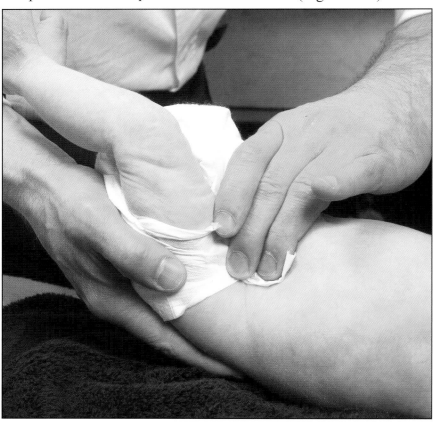

Figure 6.10 Sacral respiratory examination and correction.

THE CRANIUM

After a visual assessment of the cranium a thorough palpatory examination is indicated.

The sutures are palpated for ridging (which may indicate cranial synostosis) and overlap (excessive or incorrect moulding during the birth process).

The fontanelles, particularly the anterior and posterior fontanelles, are palpated for size and tension (Figure 6.11). (The posterior fontanelle closes at about 1 year of age and the anterior fontanelle at approximately 2 years.) Excessive tension in the fontanelles can indicate increased intracranial pressure (the baby must be relaxed as crying increases intracranial pressure), and a dipped fontanelle can indicate dehydration (a common cause of death in infants) or congenital hypothyroidism.

Any lumps or unusual shapes, such as cephalhaematoma and caput succedaneum should be palpated and assessed.

The occiput

At birth, the occiput is a composite bone made up of four parts, the basilar portion joining on to the sphenoid, the condylar or lateral portions and the squamous portion. The condylar, basilar and squamous portions are joined by a cartilaginous matrix, which is deformable. The condylar and squamous potions fuse when the child is approximately 3 years of age (Carreiro 2003).

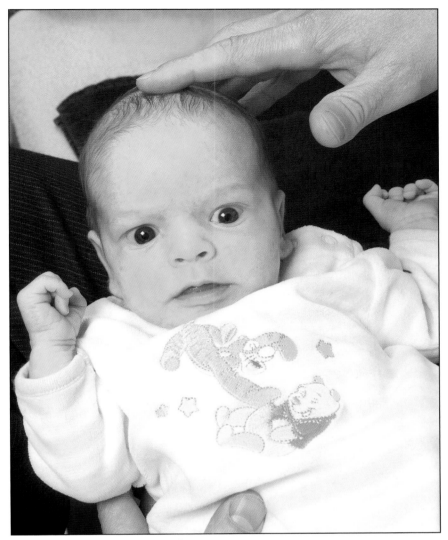

Figure 6.11 Palpation of the fontanelles.

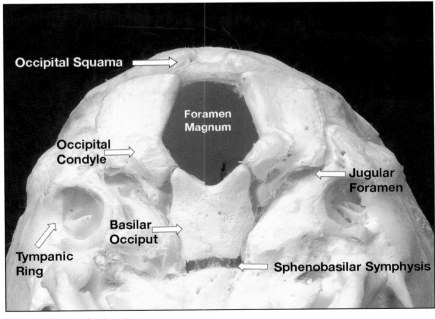

Occipital Squama

Foramen Magnum

Occipital Condyle

Jugular Foramen

Basilar Occiput

Tympanic Ring

Sphenobasilar Symphysis

Figure 6.12 Late fetal occiput.

71

Because of the ability of the fibrocartilagenous matrix to deform, the jugular foramen (between the petrous temporal bone and the condylar occiput) and the hypoglossal canals (travelling between the basilar and condylar portions of the occiput) are in particular danger of compromise (Figure 6.12). These foramina carry not only the cranial nerves, but also adipose tissue, blood vessels, connective tissue and dura, so a small degree of compromise in foramen size can potentially lead to a significant compromise of nerve function.

Assessment

The infant is laid in a supine position, preferably sucking a dummy (pacifier) or a finger; the action of sucking, as the forces are transferred through the cranium, allows stresses in the dura to be more easily palpated and corrected. The doctor contacts the infant's occiput with the fingers of both hands as near the foramen magnum as possible.

Tissue pliability is tested very gently by tractioning the tissues away from the foramen magnum, laterally and superiorly (Figure 6.13). In health, the tissues should show an even plasticity and pliability. Restrictions are more commonly unilateral but may be bilateral.

This assessment technique can easily be practised on adults before being applied to babies; it takes a short period of time for the necessary 'feel' or palpatory skill to be gained.

Correction

In this type of subtle cranial work, corrections are performed in the

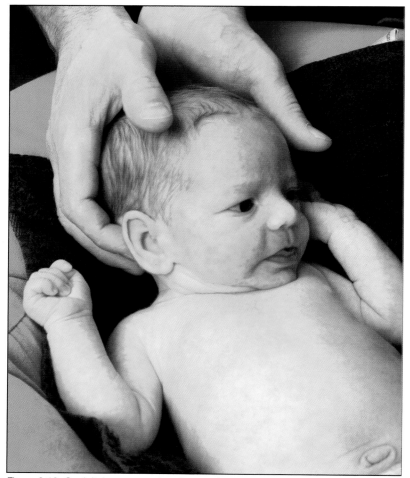

Figure 6.13 Occipital assessment and correction.

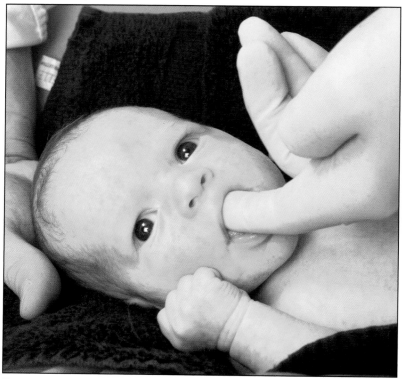

Figure 6.14 Alternative occiput correction.

direction of free motion – an indirect technique. It is a matter of following the direction of freedom out of the tissue tension. These fascial and dural restrictions are not easily freed simply by using force in the direction of correction but are better 'unwound' to gradually untangle the restrictions that have occurred. Indirect techniques are contrary to the direct adjusting techniques learnt at chiropractic college; in these, movement is imparted to a fixated vertebra with a direct adjustment into the restriction.

Becoming proficient in indirect cranial techniques takes a small change of mindset and a little practice. This is worthwhile as it opens up a whole new world of powerful therapeutic corrections.

The side of occipital restriction needs to be gently coaxed to release it. When restriction is noted, gently attempt to move the tissues laterally and follow the release. If no tissue release is apparent, try to move the tissues medially, in an oblique or rotational vector, or even further into the lesion under the occiput. One of these vectors will allow a tissue 'give'; follow this until it stops and then try all other vectors again until you can once more follow the direction of tissue release or freedom. Continue until the occiput feels pliable in all directions. The

other side may now feel more restricted in comparison to the corrected side, so release that in the same way.

The occiput may also be corrected using one hand with two fingers to either side of the occipital squama and correcting as above. The infant can then suck on a finger from the free hand (Figure 6.14).

After a lot of practice with this technique, it will gradually become apparent that there is no need to challenge all vectors to release the restrictions. The tissue unwinding will become intuitive, and your hands will just follow the vectors that lead you through the tissue restrictions.

The occipital condyle

Dejarnette, in his work *Cranial Technique (1979)*, describes a method of correction for the occipital condyles. I believe that this is primarily a test and correction for a restriction between the occipital condyle and the atlas rather than between the portions of the occiput, but it is a very useful correction.

Assessment

The infant lies supine with doctor contacting the posterior skull with eight fingers, and with his or her thumbs on the frontal bones. The head is then taken in left and right lateral flexion

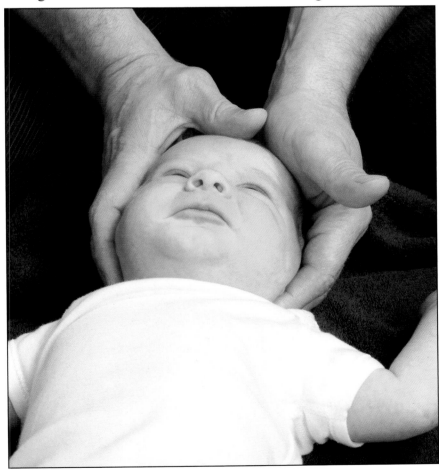

Figure 6.15 Occipital condyle assessment – left lateral flexion.

73

to assess motion (Figure 6.15). This is not full lateral flexion involving cervical motion but is just isolated to the occiput on the atlas. Any restriction of motion or hardness of end-feel is abnormal and is noted.

Correction

Occipital condyle restriction can be corrected in one of two ways: direct or indirect (Dejarnette 1979). The indirect method is the method of choice, although it might take slightly longer, as it generally seems to be more comfortable for the infant.

- *Indirect method.* The infant's skull is laterally flexed to the side of least restriction and held there. It will tend to release further into that direction; as it does, keep the skull in tight lateral flexion and follow the release. Retest the side of restriction, which should now be considerably more mobile.

- *Direct method.* The infant's cranium is taken into the side of the restriction and held there until a release occurs. Infants will often complain vigorously in this position, and this method should only be used if the indirect method has failed.

The sphenoid

Owing to the fact that the sphenoid adjoins the basocciput (fusion usually taking place in the early twenties), it is influenced by distortions of the component

parts of the occiput. Therefore if these component parts of the occiput are disturbed, lesions of the sphenobasilar symphysis and the sphenoid itself are common.

These include superior and inferior vertical strains, lateral strains, side bends and torsions, and are covered in detail in the next chapter.

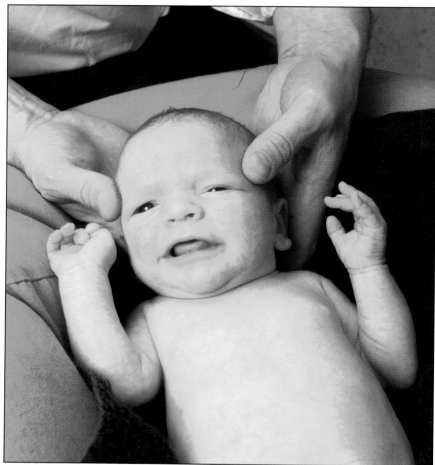

Figure 6.16 The sphenoid – bi-lateral thumb contacts.

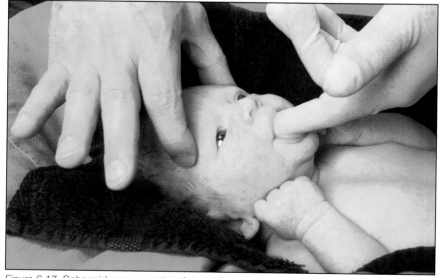

Figure 6.17 Sphenoid assessment and correction – bridge contact.

The main parts of the sphenoid that we can assess easily in infants are the greater wings, which lie just posterior to the outer canthus of the eye. They are formed in membrane so are more susceptible to trauma and distortion than bones formed from cartilage; very light contacts are therefore necessary (Figure 6.6 above).

Assessment

The sphenoid is assessed by very gently contacting the greater wings and taking them into flexion (anterior–inferior) and then into extension (posterior–superior), checking for ease of motion or restriction. This can be performed with thumb and forefinger contact and the rest of the hand bridging over the cranium. It is, however, better in my experience for those new to cranial work to contact the greater wings with the same fingers of both hands, i.e. the forefingers, middle fingers or thumbs. This is because the palpatory experience of sphenoid movement is somewhat more difficult to assess with the thumb and a finger as they have different proprioceptive qualities, and excessive compression of the infant's sphenoid by the doctor is also less likely (Figures 6.16 and 6.17).

Correction

If a restriction is noted in flexion or extension on either greater wing, motion is introduced in the direction of least resistance. For example, if the left greater wing will not easily go into flexion, take it into the direction it will go, which may be extension, superior, inferior or rotary motion, and follow its movement until a release has been completed. The greater wing should now move freely through both flexion and extension. This may be performed bilaterally if both sides are restricted.

The temporal bones

At birth, the temporal bones are in three sections: the tympanic ring, the petrous portion and the squama. The mastoid process is not developed at birth (hence the susceptibility of the facial nerve to damage in the delivery process, where it exits the stylomastoid foramen). With this in mind, the mastoid cannot be used as a lever to correct the temporal bone, as is commonly the case in the adult cranial technique. The easiest technique to use for assessment and correction is the ear pull, in which the pinna of the ear is used as a lever for correction. The fascia from the pinna is continuous around the temporal bone and into the ear canal itself.

Assessment

Grasp the pinnae of the infant's ears bilaterally and gently induce a slight lateral tension. Any restriction will easily be apparent as little lateral movement will be forthcoming (Figure 6.18).

Correction

As with the correction for the occiput and sphenoid bone, try to follow the direction of free movement of the restricted temporal bone. This may be superior, inferior, anterior,

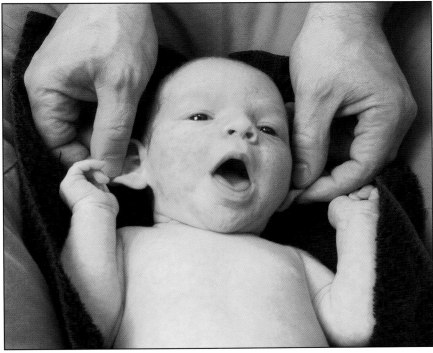

Figure 6.18 Temporal ear-pull technique.

posterior or quite commonly in a rotational direction. The free direction of movement is followed until each pinna feels pliable on gentle lateral traction.

After 3 years of age, the temporal bone can be corrected using the reciprocating temporal rocker technique (Dejarnette 1979). The mastoids are contacted with the thenar eminences, with the rest of the hands under the occiput. The doctor then very gently brings the distal ends of the thenar eminences together by flaring out his or her elbows. This causes the tips of the mastoids to approximate and the temporal bones to go into external rotation or flexion (Figure 6.19). This is then released as the doctor brings his or her elbows back into the midline, causing the mastoid tips to separate and allowing the temporal bones back into internal rotation or extension (Figure 6.20). If there is restriction, this process can be repeated a number of times until motion has been obtained or alternatively the mobile side can be held still and just the hypomobile side corrected. This is a direct technique.

If, after using either of the above techniques, good temporal motion is not accomplished, the cause is most commonly compression of the zygoma causing locking of the temporal–zygomatic suture. This is released by inserting a gloved little finger into the baby's cheek to the zy-

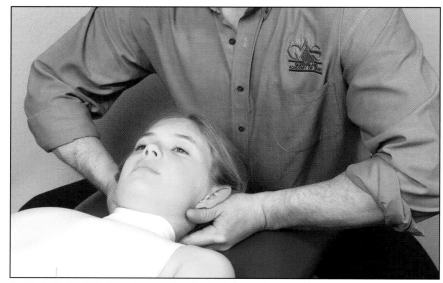

Figure 6.19 Reciprocating temporal rocker technique – temporal flexion.

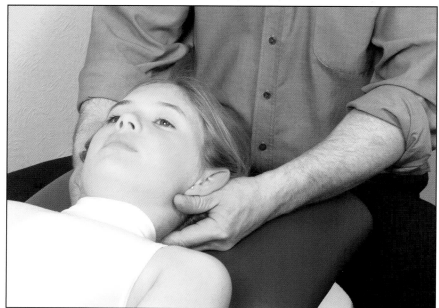

Figure 6.20 Reciprocating temporal rocker technique – temporal extension.

gomatic fossa and very gently rolling it outward and releasing any restriction in the fossa (Figure 6.24 below). Note that the tissues around the zygomatic fossa can be very sensitive so this procedure must be performed with the utmost gentleness.

The frontal bone(s)

The infant is born with a metopic suture effectively creating two frontal bones. The age of fusion of the metopic suture is variable, but this often starts around 3 months and in most cases is complete by 9 months of age (Vu et al 2001).

During the birth process, the frontal bones normally telescope under the parietal bones (Carlan et al 1991) and then remould in the hours following birth. During the birth process, one frontal bone occasionally overrides the parietal bone and gets stuck. These babies have a startled look, with one eye bigger in the superior to inferior diameter. A palpable overlap is also present where the frontal bone overrides the parietal.

More commonly, the frontal bones, if lesioned, are compressed towards the facial complex. This will tend to restrict dural movement, because of the attachments of the falx cerebri.

Assessment

With the infant supine contact the angles of the frontal bones bilaterally (just superior to the lateral border of the outer canthus of the eye) using the fore- and middle fingers; with the thumbs, contact the junction between the frontal and parietal bones either side of the anterior fontanelle. The frontal is then very gently lifted towards the ceiling (Figure 6.21). Any restriction is noted; this may be bilateral or unilateral.

The junction between the frontal and the parietal bones should also be palpated for any overlap. The metopic suture is intact in many infants up to 9 months of age so this should be examined for ridging or overlap.

An assessment of metopic motion (which is particularly important under 3 months of age) is performed by contacting either side of the metopic suture with four fingers of each hand. Shear

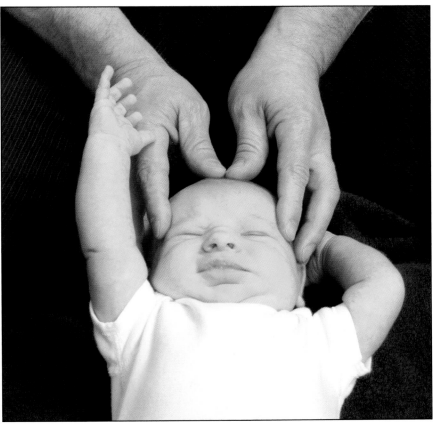

Figure 6.21 Frontal bone assessment and release.

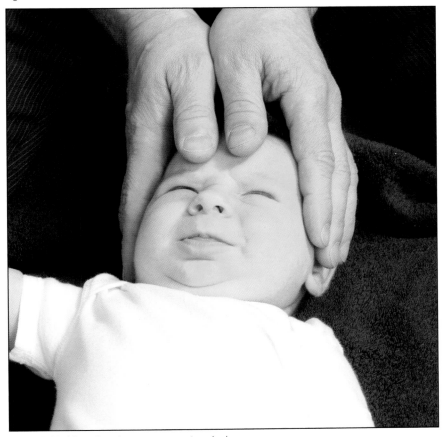

Figure 6.22 Metopic suture assessment and release.

stress is very gently assessed by lifting one side superiorly and moving inferiorly with the other. This is then repeated in the other direction and any restriction noted (Figure 6.22).

Correction

If an overlap of the frontal bone over the parietal is noted, the thumbs are placed on to the overlap as if to push the frontal bone off the parietal. The remaining fingers contact the lateral aspects of the infant's skull bilaterally. The thumbs try all directions of motion until a free motion is found (even if the motion appears to worsen the lesion), and this is followed until the movement ceases. Again, all direction of movement is tried until another free movement is found. This protocol is followed until all movements are free and the overlap has gone. This will usually take one or two applications.

When correcting frontal compression (before or after closure of the metopic suture), the hand positions are the same as for assessment, with two fingers to the frontal angles and the thumbs either side of the anterior fontanelle bilaterally. If one or both sides of the frontal bone cannot be lifted, a direction of free movement is again sought and followed until the restriction has been unwound and the frontal is pliable (contacts as in Figure 6.21). Any restriction at the metopic suture is corrected in the same fashion, following

the direction of free motion (contacts as in Figure 6.22).

The maxillae

The maxillae have little vertical development at birth and are relatively flat (Magoun 1976). A suture separates the maxillae proper from the premaxilla; this allows growth to occur anteriorly as well as laterally at the intermaxillary suture. The maxillae are particularly susceptible to trauma in face presentations and forceps deliveries, which can disrupt and distort the component parts of the hard palate.

Assessment

Visual assessment of the level of the maxillae is difficult in infants, but an uneven smile or scowl can give a clue to a non-level maxilla. Once the teeth have arrived, a pencil or tongue depressor placed behind the upper incisors can give a reasonably accurate guide to maxillary level.

Palpatory assessment is carried out with a gloved forefinger in the mouth. The intermaxillary and premaxillary sutures are palpated for ridging, distortion or overlap. The bones of the maxillae should be pliable, and any hard or restricted points are noted (Figure 6.23).

This is a good time to assess the infant's suck, which should be neither too strong nor feeble, and should have a soft rippling action of the tongue when resting between active sucking (see sucking disorders).

Correction

Any unevenness of the maxillary or premaxillary suture should be corrected first. There are a number of methods for correcting the

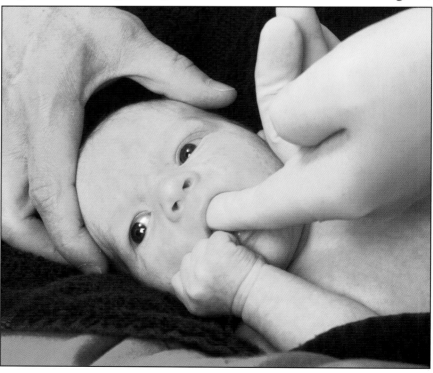

Figure 6.23 Maxillary assessment and release.

maxillae; the method described here is the method of choice for ease of use.

The forefinger lying within the mouth contacts the site of sutural distortion or any area of hard, resistant bone within the maxillae themselves. The doctor's other hand straddles the infant's frontal bone, contacting gently with thumb and forefinger on the greater wing of the sphenoid. This is then taken into flexion and extension (Figure 6.24). The finger in the mouth subtly changes the vector of the palate contact (the baby's suck aiding this gentle pressure) until a 'give' or release of the maxilla is felt as the sphenoid is mobilised.

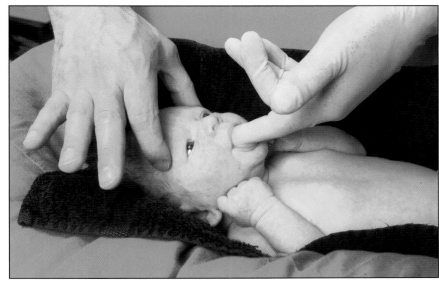

Figure 6.24 *Maxilla/sphenoid release.*

The zygoma

The zygomatic or malar bones act as keystones or locking bones for the facial complex. This is most easily demonstrated when disarticulating a skull: it is necessary to remove the zygoma to disengage the facial complex.

The zygomatic arches are strong and prominent at birth and articulate with the maxillae, the frontal bones and the temporal bones. A zygoma that is compressed can inhibit the motion of any of these bones.

Assessment

Assessment of zygomatic motion can be either internal or external. External assessment involves contacting the zygoma bilaterally with three fingers from each hand and very gently

assessing motion and play in all directions while noting the direction of any restrictions.

Assessment from within the mouth is performed individually on each zygoma using a gloved finger (if the doctor has large hands, the little finger may be the most applicable). The finger slides up laterally from the maxilla into the zygomatic fossa. This procedure should be undertaken

slowly and very gently as the fossa is very delicate and small, usually only admitting a fingertip. The finger is then rolled laterally, assessing the motion and play in the three sutures. The doctor's other hand externally palpates all three sutures as the finger in the mouth is rolled out and assesses the mobility; again any restriction and its location is noted (Figure 6.25).

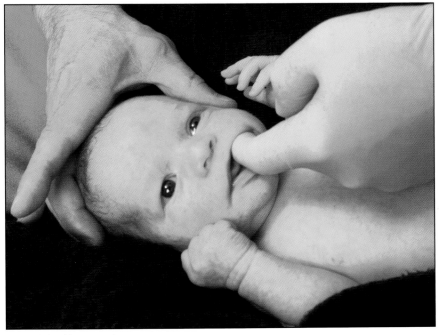

Figure 6.25 *Zygoma release.*

Correction

To correct a zygomatic compression externally, it is usually necessary to follow the direction of motion opposite to that of the restriction. The release is carried on in the direction of free motion until mobility has been established in the original direction of restriction.

To correct a zygomatic compression from within the mouth, the finger in the mouth rolls laterally into the restriction and then changes vector into any direction of free motion; this is followed with the external fingers over the involved suture(s). All directions of free motion are explored and followed until the restriction has been released and good mobility has achieved.

The nasal bones

The neonate's nasal bones are very small, each measuring only a few millimetres, and are easily subject to trauma during the birth process (Magoun 1976). The most common lesion occurs when the nasal bones are compressed up under the frontal bone; this can contribute to babies having difficulty breathing through their noses. Displacement of the nasal septum is also a relatively common trauma during birth, and the technique for correcting the nasal bones will also, if used early enough, be helpful in correcting a deviated septum.

Assessment

Because of the small size of the infant's nasal bones, it can be somewhat difficult to assess them for mobility. The easiest method is to grasp them gently in a pincer fashion and stabilise the vault of the head with the other hand. Babies generally do not enjoy this very much so it is best to be as swift as possible. Gentle inferior traction is applied, and mobility in this direction is assessed; if compression is present, no motion will be felt (Figure 6.26).

Correction

The direction of free movement is sought and then followed; this may be lateral to either side, a rotary movement or even further into compression. Free movement is followed until mobility in inferior traction has been accomplished.

The parietal bones

The two parietals are the largest bones of the infant skull and may be subject to compression or occasionally overlap during

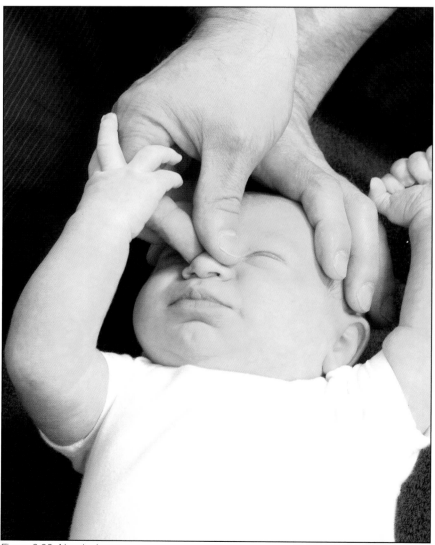

Figure 6.26 Nasal release.

the birth process. The parietal bones generally lock together at the sagittal suture during the birth process to protect the delicate tissues of the cerebral hemispheres (Carlan et al 1991), but excessive moulding occasionally occurs and some overlap may be present. They are particularly subject to stress and trauma during instrumental vaginal deliveries and are common sites for cephalhaematomas and caput succedaneum.

Assessment

The borders of each parietal bone at the sutures should be palpated for overlap. To assess mobility, the parietal bones are gently contacted by all four fingers of each hand, and subtle traction is applied. This traction is then linked with an anterior and then posterior stress to assess whether any motion is present. The direction of any restriction is noted (Figure 6.27).

'Baby hypnosis'

Figure 6.27 shows an abacus, which is used to quieten a fractious or irritable baby. The abacus is held within the baby's vision and is slowly and rhythmically tipped from side to side. The noise of the wooden beads, the colours (the abacus must be bright) and the slow cadence seem to lull most babies into a relaxed state, making treatment much easier.

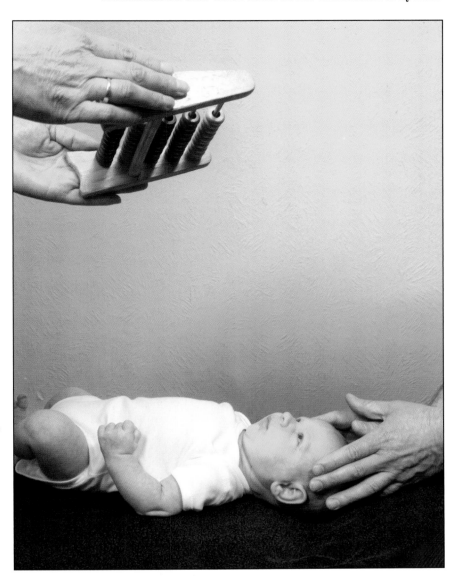

Figure 6.27 Parietal lift: 'baby hypnosis'.

Correction

The parietal bones are corrected with the same contacts as in the assessment, but instead of going into the direction of restriction, the direction of free motion is followed until mobility has been established. As with most of the previously discussed cranial corrections, it is a question of 'unwinding' the tissues following the path of least resistance or free motion.

81

REFERENCES

Adams T, Heisley R, Smith M, Briner B. Parietal bone mobility in the anesthetised cat. *J Am Osteopat Assoc* 1992; 92: 599–622.

Arbuckle BE. *The Selected Works of Beryl E Arbuckle*. Indianapolis: American Academy of Osteopathy, 1994.

Carlan SJ, Wyble L, Lense J, Mastrogiannis DS, Parsons MT. Fetal head moulding. Diagnosis by ultrasound and a review of the literature. *J Perinatal* 1991; 11: 105–111.

Carreiro JE. *An Osteopathic Approach to Children*. Edinburgh: Churchill Livingstone, 2003.

Chaitow L. *Cranial Manipulation Theory and Practice*. Edinburgh: Churchill Livingstone, 1999.

Degenhardt B, Kuchera M. Update on osteopathic medical concepts and the lymphatic system. *J Am Osteopat Assoc* 1996; 96: 97–100.

DeJarnette MB. *Cranial Technique*. Private publication, Nebraska City, USA, 1979.

Gehin A. *Atlas of Manipulative Techniques for the Cranium and Face*. Seattle: Eastland Press, 1985.

Feinberg DA, Mark AS. Human brain motion and cerebral spinal fluid circulation demonstrated with MR velocity imaging. *Radiology* 1987; 163: 793–799.

Ferguson A. Cranial osteopathy: a new perspective. *Acad Appl Osteopat J* 1991; 4:12–16.

Heisey S, Adams T. Role of cranial bone mobility in cranial compliance. *Neurosurgery* 1993; 33: 869–877.

Howat JMP. *The Anatomy and Physiology of Sacro Occipital Technique*. Private publication, Oxford, 1999.

Lewandoski M, Drasby E. Kinematic system demonstrates cranial bone movement about the cranial suture. *J Am Osteopat Assoc* 1996; 96: 551.

Lewer Allen K, Bunt E. Dysfunctioning of fluid mechanical craniospinal systems as revealed by stress/strain diagrams. Presentation to the International Conference on Bio Engineering and Biophysics, Jerusalem 1979. Reported in: Upledger J. *Research Supports Existence of Craniosacral System*. Palm Beach, Florida: Upledger Institute Enterprises, 1979.

Lumsden C. Normal oligodendrocytes in tissue culture. *Exp Cell Res* 1951; 2: 103–114.

McPartland J, Mein E. Entrainment and the cranial rhythmic impulse. *Altern Ther Health Med* 1997; 3: 40–44.

Magoun HI. *Osteopathy in the Cranial Field*. Boise, Idaho: Cranial Academy, 1976.

Pederick FO. A Kaminski-type evaluation of cranial adjusting. *Chiropr Tech* 1997; 9(1).

Podlas H, Lewer Allen K, Bunt E. Computed tomography studies of human brain movements. *S Afr J Surg* 1984; 22: 57–63.

Sutherland W. *The Cranial Bowl*. Mankato, Minnesota: Free Press, 1939.

Tettambal M, Cicoea R, Lay E. Recording of cranial rhythmic impulse. *J Am Osteopat Assoc* 1978; 78: 149.

Upledger JE. *A Brain is Born*. Berkley, California: North Atlantic Books, 1996.

Upledger JE, Vredevoogd JD. *Craniosacral Therapy*. Seattle: Eastland Press, 1983.

Vu HL, Panchal J, Parker EE, Levine NS, Francel P. The timing of physiolgic closure of the metopic suture: a review of 159 patients using reconstructed 3D CT scans of the craniofacial region. *J Craniofac Surg* 2001; 12: 527–532 .

Illustrations in Chapter Six

Examination and correction of the craniosacral system

Chapter 7
Plagiocephaly

The term 'plagiocephaly' is derived from the Greek words meaning oblique head. Glat et al (1996) classified plagiocephaly into three main types:

- type 1 – from cranial suture synostosis;
- type 2 – from non-synostotic causes (deformational);
- type 3 – from craniofacial microsomia-associated plagiocephaly.

For the purposes of this chapter, we will concentrate on types 1 and 2: synostotic plagiocephaly and non-synostotic deformational plagiocephaly (NSDP).

Synostotic plagiocephaly arises as a result of so called premature sutural fusion. One may take issue with the term 'premature' as the fusion of most cranial sutures is abnormal. Craniosynostotic plagiocephaly results from the growing brain compressing the skull, which cannot expand normally because of fusion of the sutures.

The shape of the skull will depend on where the sutural fusion occurs. For example, fusion of the sagittal suture will lead to scaphocephaly or a very long, thin, narrow head. Fusion unilaterally of one lambdoid suture will give a trapezoid-shaped head with flattening of the ipsilateral side of the back of the skull. Fusion of a coronal suture unilaterally will have the same effect on the front of the skull, excluding the face.

The aetiology of craniosynostosis is unknown, but theories have been put forward linking it to fetal head constraint (Graham et al 1980, Higginbottom et al 1980). In murine (mice) studies, Kirschner et al (2002) demonstrated the ability of intrauterine constraint (in this case artificially induced) to produce cranial asymmetry and sutural fusion. More research is, however, needed before we can talk with any certainty of constraint being the cause of synostotic plagiocephaly.

NSDP has also been termed positional plagiocephaly (Clarren 1981) in reference to the supposed cause: the baby's sleeping or lying position. Boere-Boonekamp and van der Linden-Kuiper (2001) screened over 6000 infants for what they termed positional preference (the infant turning his or her head to one side most of the time) and found it to be present in 8.2% of babies. Of these, 42% showed asymmetrical occipital flattening and 23% asymmetrical frontal flattening. The 8.2% of children with positional preference may well have been suffering from kinematic imbalances due to suboccipital strain (KISS) syndrome, of which common features incliude positional preference and plagiocephaly (Biedermann 2005).

Peitsch et al (2002), in a cross-sectional study of healthy neonates, found the incidence of anomalous head shapes in single-born infants to be 24% and in twins 56%. The risk factors they identified were assisted vaginal delivery, primiparity, prolonged labour, unusual birth position and male gender. They proposed that the head flattening they observed at birth was a precursor to plagiocephaly, particularly associated with a supine sleeping position, and proposed the use of alternate sleeping postures (side, back, side).

The developmental outcomes of children with NSDP were looked at by Miller and Clarren (2000); 39.7% of children with NSDP in the study received special help in primary school, and the authors concluded that children with NSDP comprised a high-risk group for developmental difficulties.

DIFFERENTIAL DIAGNOSIS

Cervical ranges of motion and palpation of the sternocleidomastoid muscles should always be undertaken to rule out the possibility of plagiocephaly secondary to a sternocleidomastoid torticollis.

The importance of a differential diagnosis between synostotic plagiocephaly and NSDP is vital for providing a conservative treatment prognosis and for assessing the need for early surgical intervention.

Bony ridging or peaking is commonly noted in metopic and sagittal synostosis, but it is less predictive in unilaterally coronal or lambdoidal synostosis (Bruneteau and Mulliken 1992). Radiographic studies of the skull can be diagnostic in advanced cases of synostosis, but early signs can be very difficult to detect (Bruneteau and Mulliken 1992). Computerised tomography and magnetic resonance imaging are the methods of choice for the diagnosis of synostosis, but they require the baby to be anaesthetised and should be used only when there is a significant suspicion of synostosis.

The major difficulty lies in the differential diagnosis between unilateral coronal synostosis and NSDP at the anterior skull, and unilateral lambdoidal synostosis and NSDP at the posterior skull.

Unilateral coronal synostosis versus NSDP

Bruneteau and Mulliken (1992) used cranial landmarks as part of a useful methodology for the differential diagnosis of frontal plagiocephaly. Specifically, when viewed from the vertex, the side of frontal flattening will tend to have an anterior displacement of the ipsilateral ear and sparing of the face in unilateral coronal synostosis. NSDP will tend to have a posteriorly displaced ear on the side of frontal flattening and facial mirroring of the flattened frontal bone (Figure 7.1).

Unilateral lambdoidal synostosis versus NSDP

In a clinical guidance bulletin, the American Academy of Paediatrics (2003) recommended that if the unilateral occipital flattening was present at birth, a diagnosis of lambdoidal synostosis should be considered, and if the flattening began a few weeks afterwards, the diagnosis was probably NSDP.

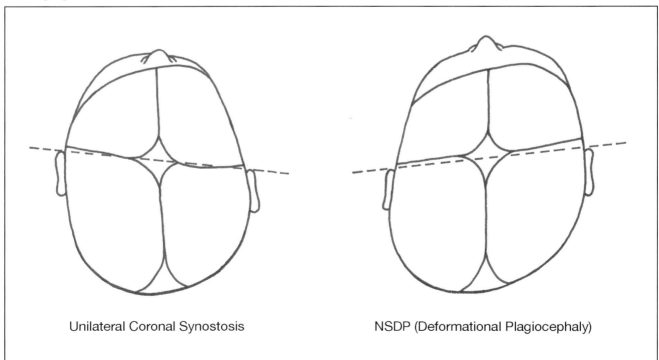

Unilateral Coronal Synostosis   NSDP (Deformational Plagiocephaly)

Figure 7.1 Unilateral coronal synostosis versus non-synostotic deformational plagiocephaly (NSDP).

They further suggested a number of physical signs to differentiate lambdoidal synostosis and NSDP. Specifically, with lambdoidal synostosis, the ear ipsilateral to the side of occipital flattening was typically posterior compared with the contralateral ear, whereas in deformational posterior plagiocephaly, the ipsilateral ear was anterior on the side of skull flattening (Figure 7.2).

Referral for advanced imaging should always be made when there is a suspicion of synostosis. Surgery is usually indicated in cases of synostosis to avoid a restriction of vault growth and impairment of brain development (Carriero 2003). Postsurgical chiropractic cranial evaluation is recommended, but it is generally advisable to wait for 2–3 months after surgery.

Non-synostotic deformational plagiocephaly

NSDP covers a number of different skull strain patterns, which will be covered in detail later in this chapter. It can occur secondary to a congenital muscular torticollis or from abnormal positioning. This can happen when the child lies supine with the head resting predominantly on one side of the occiput. It is, however, commonly present as a result of intrauterine constraint.

Children born vaginally will often not exhibit a skull strain pattern at birth but will develop one a few weeks later, and it is interesting to speculate on the reasons for this. Arbuckle (1994), in her writings on the

oblique skull, discussed how the trapezoid deformity of the vault of the skull was the result of a deformation of the cartilaginous base, particularly the component parts of the occiput.

It seems likely, when an infant is born with a seemingly symmetrical vault that a few weeks later becomes misshapen, that there was a disturbance of the cartilaginous portions of the skull base in utero. Owing to cranial moulding during birth, this is not, however, reflected in the skull vault. Over the weeks after birth, the action of the dura pulling on the skull vault with an uneven stress caused by distortion of the skull base then produces a vault distortion in the first weeks of rapid growth. A uniform sleeping position will of course aggravate this. The

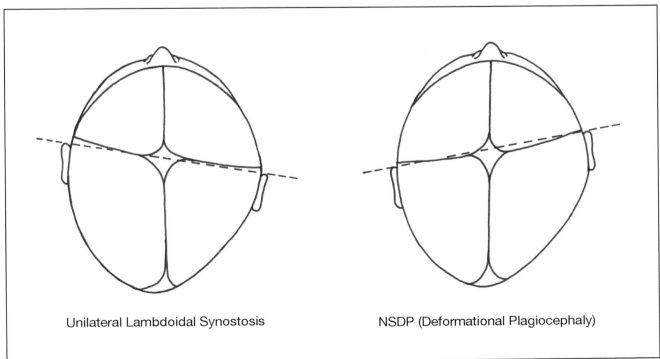

Unilateral Lambdoidal Synostosis   NSDP (Deformational Plagiocephaly)

Figure 7.2 Unilateral lambdoidal synostosis versus non-synostotic deformational plagiocephaly (NSDP).

Plagiocephaly

type of skull base disruption will often specify the shape of the vault distortion, which aids in our visual diagnosis of the lesion and therefore subsequent treatment protocols.

Arbuckle (1994) postulated that what she termed 'stress fibres' in the dura would distort the skull vault when the skull base, particularly the occiput, was disrupted. She stated that these stress fibres were both protective, deflecting the stress of excessive cranial moulding, and also had the potential to cause skull strains when the skull base was distorted.

Davies (2002) produced an interesting study involving the chiropractic management of 25 cases of deformational plagiocephaly, with a satisfactory resolution of the condition in all cases.

SKULL STRAIN PATTERNS AND CORRECTIONS

When analysing the skull for strain patterns, it is necessary to think three-dimensionally rather than in terms of a flat plane. It is also important to have a sound knowledge of cranial anatomy. The cranium is capable of pivoting at two junctions in the horizontal plane: the sphenobasilar symphysis, and the junction of the maxilla and the sphenoid bones (including the palatines in between). This allows us to analyse the skull

in three sections; the posterior part (comprising the occiput and temporal bones), the central part (the sphenoid and frontal bones) and the anterior part (the maxilla and facial complex).

Walker (1996) developed an analytical technique called triplanar analysis to analyse the various compartmental planes of the skull. The landmarks he used in older children and adults for analysis in the horizontal plane are the ears (temporal bones and occiput), eyes (sphenoid bones) and first upper premolars (maxilla) (Figure 7.3). To perform a triplanar analysis, the doctor places his or her forefingers in the patient's ear canals, positioning them parallel to the floor. The doctor's thumbs are placed on the orbital notches on the lat-

eral orbital rim, and the distances between the horizontal planes of the fingers and thumbs are analysed. This provides an assessment of any torsion between the sphenoid and the occiput.

A pencil or tongue depressor placed behind the upper canine teeth will also show the level of the maxilla. This is then compared with the level of the sphenoid, any torsion between the sphenoid and maxilla then being apparent. In the case of children and babies too young to have canine teeth, an estimation of maxillary level can be gained by observation and palpation within the mouth. A significant maxillary distortion in a baby is demonstrated by an uneven smile or scowl, the high side of the mouth reflecting the high maxilla.

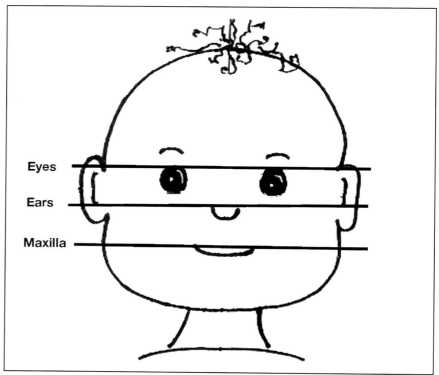

Figure 7.3 Triplanar analysis.

This procedure gives us a method of analysing the relative torsions between the front, middle and posterior elements of the skull. However, as well as analysing the skull in the anterior–posterior direction, it is very important to view the skull from the vertex down. The analysis should include the following:

- *The relative width and length of the skull.* Is it wide and short – flexion pattern. Is it long and narrow – extension pattern? Is it wide at the front and narrow at the back – superior vertical strain? Is it narrow at the front and wide at the back – inferior vertical strain?

- *The position of the nose.* Is it central and in line with the anterior and posterior fontanelles? Are the fontanelles themselves in the central line of the skull?

- *Are the ears in line across the skull,* or does one lie more anteriorly than the other?

- *Is the skull a symmetrical oval shape?* Are there any flattened areas at the anterior or posterior or both?

These questions are just a checklist that will become automatic with practice. Their job is to tell the doctor whether or not a skull strain is present, and if one is, whether it fits into any of the common skull strain patterns.

Flexion strain

A flexion strain occurs when the skull is narrowed in the anterior–posterior diameter and widened in the transverse diameter. The skull is, however, symmetrical, with the ears in the same plane across the skull and the nose in line with the fontanelles. Flexion strains tend to produce flat and widened facial features, ears that stick out from the skull and a flat occiput. They are aggravated by constantly placing a baby to sleep supine. The sphenobasilar symphysis is in flexion, with a flexed occiput, sphenoid bone and maxillae (Figures 7.4a and 7.4b).

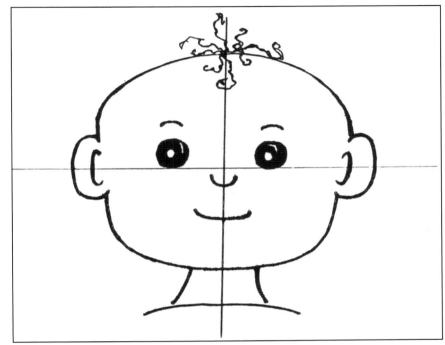
Figure 7.4a Flexion strain: anterior view.

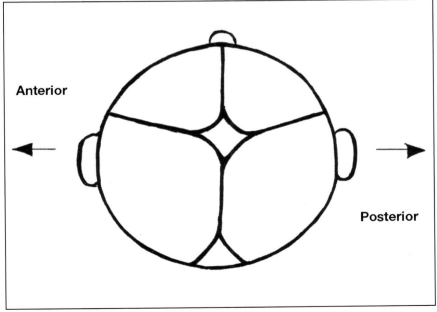
Figure 7.4b Flexion strain: vertex view.

Plagiocephaly

Correction

The occipital squama is gently contacted with one hand by the doctor on its lateral borders, with the thumb and curled forefinger just medial to the occipital mastoid suture. The greater wings of the sphenoid are contacted by the doctor's other hand, the thumb and forefinger bridging over the frontal bones. The occiput and sphenoid are taken very gently into extension; the occiput is squeezed gently and the sphenoid greater wings are taken posterior–superior (back and up).

The adjustment is made by a finger (of an assistant or parent) within the mouth contacting the anterior maxilla and lifting

gently to the vertex. This lift tensions the posterior edge of the vomer and extends the sphenoid and ethmoid, which activates the intercranial dural membrane system to assist the correction (Figure 7.5). The doctor may need to instruct the assistant to change the vectors slightly (more anterior/superior/posterior) until a give or release is felt.

The adjustment may need repeating on several visits. The skull shape should show some improvement, and there should be a significant improvement in function.

Extension strain

An extension strain occurs when the anterior/posterior diameter is lengthened and the transverse

diameter narrowed. The skull is, however, symmetrical when viewed from the vertex, with the ears in the same transverse plane and the nose in line with the fontanelles. Extension strains tend to produce long narrow facial features, with the ears flat to the skull and a narrow occiput. The sphenobasilar symphysis is in extension, with an extended occiput, sphenoid and maxilla (Figure 7.6a and 7.6b).

Correction

The occiput is contacted with one hand by the doctor, with the forefinger transverse across the nuchal line of the occiput. The greater wings of the sphenoid are contacted by the doctor's other hand, the thumb and forefinger bridging over the frontal bone. The occiput and sphenoid are very gently taken into flexion; the doctor's forefinger gently lifts the lower occipital squama at the nuccal line towards the nose and the sphenoid's greater wings are taken into flexion (forward and down).

The adjustment is made by an finger (of an assistant or parent) within the mouth, which contacts the posterior hard palate and lifts gently. This tensions the anterior border of the vomer and brings the sphenoid and ethmoid into flexion, which activates the intracranial dural membrane system to assist the correction (Figure 7.7). The doctor may

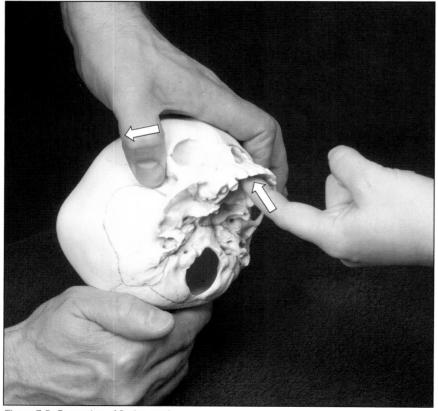

Figure 7.5 Correction of flexion strain.

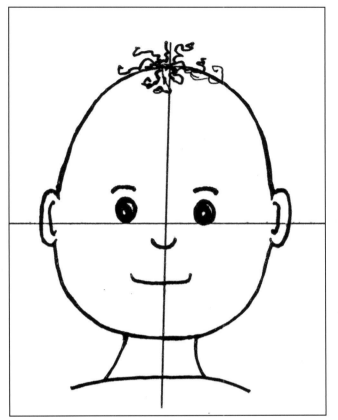

Figure 7.6a Extension strain: anterior view.

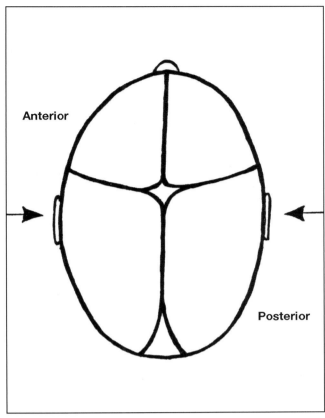

Figure 7.6b Extension strain: vertex view.

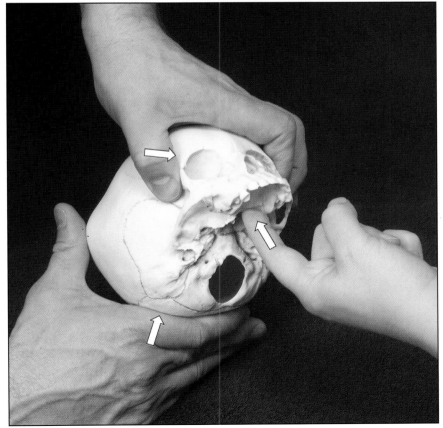

Figure 7.7 Correction of an extension strain.

need to instruct the assistant to change the vector slightly (more anterior/posterior/superior) until a give or release is felt. The adjustment may need repeating on several visits. The skull shape should show some improvement and there should be a significant improvement in skull function.

Vertical strains

These strains were first described by Sutherland and are very well documented by Magoun (1976). They represent a strain at the sphenobasilar symphysis, with the sphenoid and occiput in opposite patterns of flexion and extension. The term 'vertical strain' is used as there is a vertical shear strain through the sphenobasilar symphysis.

Plagiocephaly

Upledger and Vredevoogd (1983) state that it is common for vertical strain patterns to have a traumatic origin. This is often the case when a suction cap or forceps has been used, occiput posterior presentations being the main predisposing factor. In severe vertical strain patterns, Upledger and Vredevoogd (1983) observed that common symptoms on presentation included severe head pain, sinusitis, allergies and personality disorders.

Inferior vertical strain

An inferior vertical strain creates a flexed occiput with a wide posterior skull, and an extended sphenoid with a narrow anterior skull (Figure 7.8a and 7.8b). If severe and left untreated, it will have far-reaching consequences in the future. A marked occipital flexion will cause external rotation of the temporal bones, leading the mandibular fossa to migrate posteriorly, which induces mandibular retrusion. This mandibular retrusion generally leads to an anterior head carriage (to allow easier phonation and breathing), which often causes an increased thoracic kyphosis and lumbar lordosis, with an anterior rotation of the pelvis (sway-back posture).

As well as poor posture, children and adults with an inferior vertical strain will often exhibit a dental class I, division II bite (overbite and overjet of the

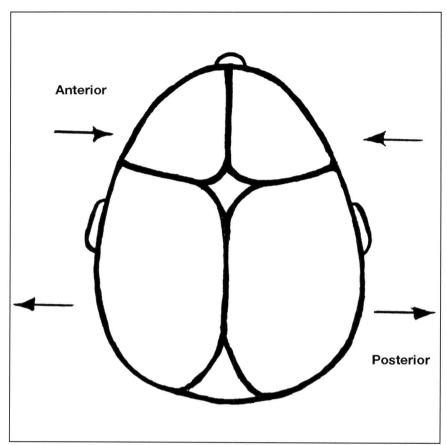

Figure 7.8a Inferior vertical strain: vertex view.

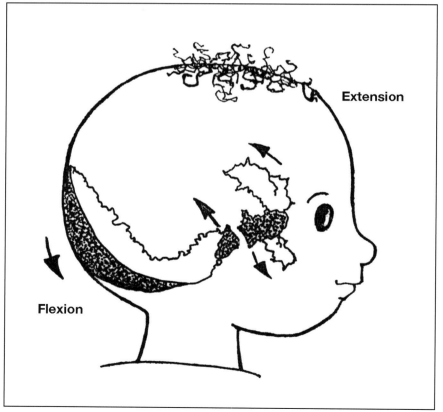

Figure 7.8b Inferior vertical strain: lateral view.

92

upper incisors with a narrow and high maxillary arch). We rarely see this dental pattern in young adults today because modern dental orthodontics usually intervene in the early teenage years. All too often, however, extraction orthodontics are undertaken, as the upper arch tends to be overcrowded, or more accurately too small for the correct number of teeth. This procedure worsens the tightness and restriction of the maxilla and predisposes towards poor sinus drainage and perhaps even poor pituitary function.

Correction. The occipital squama is contacted with one hand by the doctor on its lateral borders, with a thumb and curled forefinger just medial to the occipitomastoid suture. The sphenoid is contacted by the doctor's other hand, the thumb and forefinger bridging over the frontal bone. The occiput is then taken into extension (squeezed gently) and the sphenoid into flexion (down and forwards).

The adjustment is made by a finger (of an assistant or parent) within the mouth contacting the posterior hard palate and lifting gently. This will tension the anterior border of the vomer, bringing the sphenoid and ethmoid into flexion, and activating the cranial dural membrane system to assist the correction (Figure 7.9).

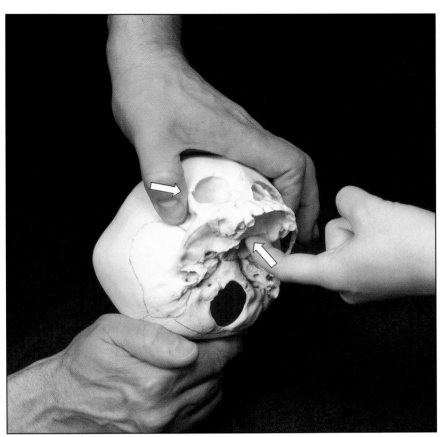

Figure 7.9 Correction of an inferior vertical strain.

Superior vertical strain

A superior vertical strain creates a flexed sphenoid, so the anterior skull is wide, and an extended occiput, so the posterior skull is narrow (Figure 7.10a and 7.10b). If the strain is severe and uncorrected, it will, as with the inferior vertical strain, have far-reaching consequences, but they will differ in character.

Occipital extension, in the presence of anterior skull flexion, causes internal rotation of the temporal bones, which moves the mandibular fossa anteriorly, leading a class III dental malocclusion (protruding jaw). The upper arch will tend be wide and flat, with flexion of the sphenoid creating maxillary flexion. These individuals often exhibit a ramrod military style posture with a loss of cervical lordosis. In my experience, probably because of the sphenoid and facial complex being stuck in flexion, individuals often exhibit a chronic postnasal drip.

Correction. The doctor contacts the occiput with one finger running across the nuchal line. The other hand bridges over the frontal bone to contact the greater wings of the sphenoid. The occiput is taken into flexion by using anterior pressure on the nuchal line towards the nose, and simultaneously the sphenoid wings are taken posterior, and superior into extension.

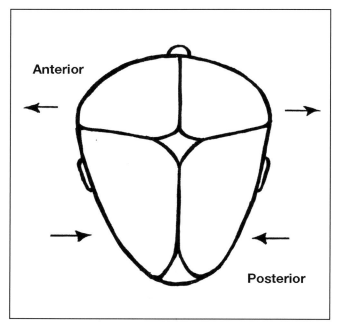

Figure 7.10a Superior vertical strain: vertex view.

Figure 7.10b Superior vertical strain: lateral view.

The adjustment is made by an assistant (or parent) contacting the anterior hard palate and lifting gently. This tensions the posterior edge of the vomer, creating extension in the sphenoid and ethmoid bones, and activation of the dural membrane system to assist the correction (Figure 7.11).

Anterior–posterior strain

This is also known as a parallelogram head or oblique skull. Obliquity of the skull was described by Little as far back as 1862 as flattening of one side of the face and the opposite side of the skull. Arbuckle (1994) stated that this shape was the result of fetal position (intrauterine constraint) in the latter stages of pregnancy.

The primary lesion, which causes this strain pattern, is a disruption of the component parts of the

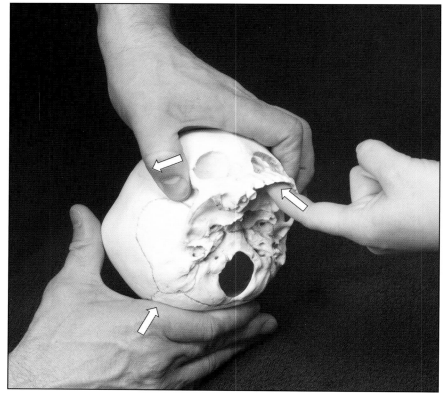

Figure 7.11 Correction of a superior vertical strain.

neonatal occiput. One condylar portion is driven anteriorly relative to the other (possibly created by an asynclistic position with some cervical extension), which will distort the basilar portion and therefore the sphenobasilar symphysis.

An interesting phenomenon is that the infant is often born with a fairly symmetrically

18 Months	over. Shows preference for one hand. Gets up/down stairs holding onto rail. Begins to jump with both feet. Can build a tower of 3 or 4 cubes and throw a ball.	mothering. Drinks from a cup with both hands. Feeds self with a spoon. Attains bowel control. Tries to sing. Imitates domestic activities.	picture books. Explores environment. Knows the names of parts of his body.	Uses many intelligible words. Repeats an adult's last word. Jabbering established.
2 Years	Can kick large ball. Squats with ease. Rises without using hands. Builds tower of six cubes. Able to run. Walks up and down stairs 2 feet per step. Builds tower of 6 cubes. Turns picture book pages one at a time.	Throws tantrum if frustrated. Can put on shoes. Completely spoon feeds and drinks from cup. Is aware of physical needs. Dry by day.	Joins 2-3 words in sentences. Recognises details in pictures. Uses own name to refer to self.	Talks to self continuously. Speaks over two hundred words, and accumulate new words very rapidly.
3 Years	Can jump off lower steps. Can pedal and steer tricycle. Goes up stairs 1 foot per step and downstairs 2 feet per step. Copies circle. Imitates cross and draws man on request. Builds tower of 9 cubes. Has good pencil control. Can cut paper with scissors. Can thread large beads on a string.	Plays co-operatively . Undresses with assistance. Imaginary companions.Tries very hard to please. Uses spoon and fork.	Relates present activities and past experiences. Can draw a person with a head. Can sort objects into simple categories.	Constantly asks questions. Speaks in sentences. Talks to himself when playing.
4 Years	Sits with knees crossed. Ball games skill increases. Goes down stairs one foot per step. Imitates gate with cubes. Copies a cross. Can turn sharp corners when running. Builds a tower of 10 cubes.	Argues with other children. Plans games co-operatively. Dresses and undresses with assistance. Attends to own toilet needs. Developing a sense of humour. Wants to be independent.	Counts up to 20. Asks meanings of words. Questioning at its height. Draw recognisable house.	Many infantile substitutions in speech. Uses correct grammar most of the time. Enjoy counting up to twenty by repetition.
5 Years	Skips. Well developed ball skills. Can walk on along a thin line. Skips on both feet and hops. Draws a man and copies a triangle. Gives age. Can copy an adult's writing. Colours pictures carefully. Builds steps with 3-4 cubes.	Chooses own friends. Dresses and undresses alone. Shows caring attitudes towards others. Copes well with personal needs.	Writes name. Draws a detailed person. Matches most colours. Understands numbers.	Fluent speech with few infantile substitutions in speech. Talks about the past, present and future with a good sense of time.
6 Years	Learns to skip with rope. Copies a diamond. Knows right from left and number of fingers. Ties shoe laces.	Stubborn and demanding. Eager for fresh experiences. May be quarrelsome with friends.	Draws with precision and to detail. Developing reading skills well. May write independently.	Fluent speech. Can pronounce majority of the sounds of his own language. Talk fluently and with confidence.

shaped skull vault and gradually demonstrates the obliquity of the skull in the following weeks and months. This is probably because, although the cranial base is distorted, the vault of the skull, having gone through the skull-moulding process during birth, appears symmetrical. During the first few weeks after birth, the vault expands and responds to the stresses imparted by the dural membrane system, which is in turn influenced by the skull base. This then results in the skull obliquity.

Viewed from the vertex, the skull shows an oblique shape (Figure 7.12a), but when viewed from the anterior, it appears to be in flexion on the anterior forehead side (wider eye and flared ear) and in extension on the posterior forehead side (narrower eye and flat ear) (Figure 7.12b).

If the infant is placed supine, as has been the recommendation for the past decade, this will tend to increase the occipital flattening, compounding the skull base strain as the infant will favour lying on the flattened occiput side, which will aggravate the strain. This drives the already anterior condylar portion of the occiput further forward.

As they develop, children with anterior–posterior strain will tend to show a unilateral cross-bite. This skull strain is the most commonly seen in practice, possibly because the obvious vault distortion creates parental concern; it has even led to the development of a cranial orthosis (helmet band) in the USA for its correction (Kelly et al 1999).

Long-term effects, not withstanding the cosmetic concerns, include the development of spinal scoliosis (Magoun 1976, Arbuckle 1994) and learning difficulties (Miller and Clarren 2000). The latter study also found that 40% of children with plagiocephaly needed remedial help in school with their learning and motor functions.

Correction

Because the vault of the neonatal skull is largely membranous in origin and the cartilaginous base is difficult to access, a method of correction had to be established that would not compromise the delicate vault tissues. This has been accomplished by using the frontal bone(s) on the lateral, superior edge of the orbit and the temporal bones just posterior to the external auditory meatus for the correction. These areas are more stable and resistant to deformation than the rest of the vault and are useful as levers.

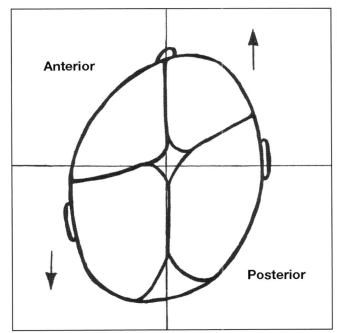

Figure 7.12a Anterior–posterior strain: vertex view.

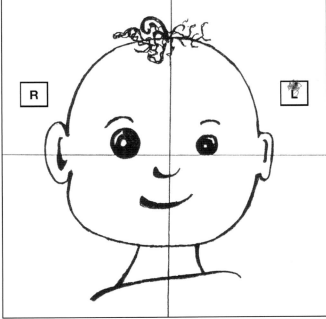

Figure 7.12b Anterior–posterior strain: anterior view.

Plagiocephaly

A contact is taken, with the lateral border of the doctor's thumb on the prominent side of the infant's frontal bone. The doctor's index finger of the same hand contacts the temporal bone just posterior to the infant's external auditory meatus. The direction of correction with this hand is posterior. The doctor's other hand, on the infant's flattened face side, contacts the temporal bone just posterior to the external auditory meatus with their forefinger. The direction of correction of this hand is anterior; this creates a sheer stress within the skull base.

The adjustment is made by having an assistant (or parent) contact the infant's maxilla with a gloved finger within the mouth on the side of the face that is flattened. The direction of correction for the contact within the mouth is anterior, with a slight lateral pull away from the flattened face (Figure 7.13). As the adjustment is performed, the doctor may need to ask the assistant to change the vector slightly laterally, medially or anteriorly. The adjustment is complete when the doctor feels a tissue 'give' or release.

Several applications may be needed, and the degree of correction may be variable. Genetic factors seem to be important in this strain pattern so check the parent's skull shape: if similar distortions are evident, the prognosis should be modified.

Lateral strain

The lateral strain is usually post-traumatic in origin (Upledger and Vredevoogd 1983), as a result of either birth trauma or head injury. Frymann (1998) reasoned that it was often caused by unilateral occipital compression during the descent of the head in the birth canal. Frymann also postulated that, after infancy, the most likely cause was trauma from a unilateral blow to the greater wings or lateral angles of the frontal bone, anterior to the vertical axis of rotation of the sphenoid.

The lesion is a lateral sheer at the sphenobasilar symphysis, with the basiocciput sheering to one side and the sphenoid body to the opposite side. Visual recognition can be slightly challenging because the jaw, the most anterior part of the cranial complex, follows the most posterior part of the skull, the occiput. This occurs because the temporal bones where the mandibular fossae are located have a close relationship with the occiput and tend to follow its strain pattern.

Viewed from above, the anterior skull shows a shift to one side and the posterior skull a shift to the opposite side (Figure 7.14a).

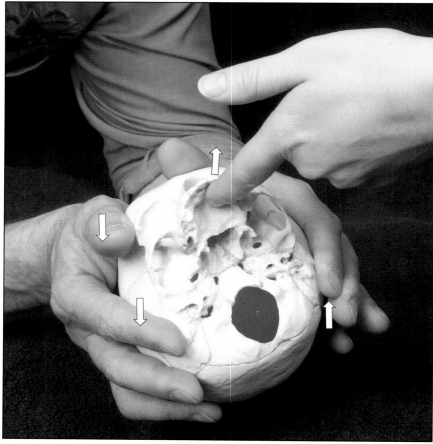

Figure 7.13 Correction of anterior–posterior strain (oblique skull).

Viewed from the anterior, the forehead will bulge on one side, with a lateral shift of the eyes to that side following the sphenoid. The jaw will be shifted across to the opposite side, creating a bilateral cross-bite in older children (Figure 7.14b). This can at times be confused with an anterior–posterior strain (and it is indeed not uncommon to have elements of both strains in a single skull), but viewing the face will give the necessary diagnostic clue to the major strain present.

An interesting additional effect of the strain was noted by Walker (1996). He found that all the adults with a lateral strain whom he had examined also had asymmetrical lower lumbar facet joints. It is interesting to speculate whether this is coincidence or a lower body adaptation to the lateral shift of the sphenoid in a lateral strain.

In my experience, many infants with lateral strains are highly symptomatic, in particular often exhibiting eye problems. Upledger and Vredevoogd (1983) noted that they had corrected many cases of strabismus in children with a lateral strain by cranial correction aimed particularly at releasing the tension in the tentorium cerebelli.

Correction

The doctor cradles the occiput with one hand, the other hand

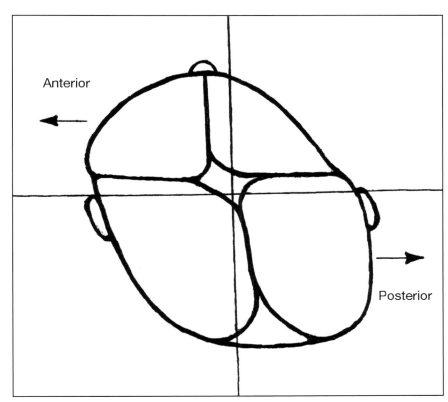

Figure 7.14a Lateral strain: vertex view.

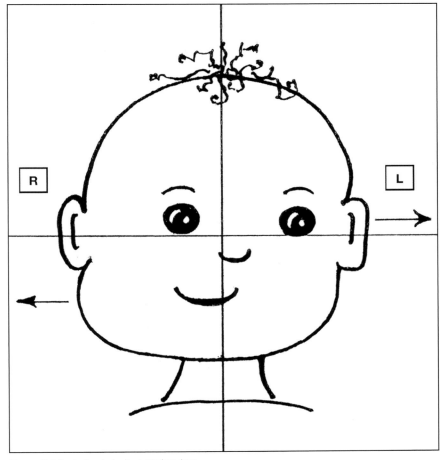

Figure 7.14b Lateral strain: anterior view.

bridging over the frontal bone to grasp the greater wings of the sphenoid. To create some sheer stress at the sphenobasilar symphysis, the occiput is gently squeezed into extension and the sphenoid wings are taken in an anterior–inferior direction into flexion. A lateral sheer is then introduced, taking the sphenoid across into correction from the side of the bulging forehead and the occiput from the bulging occiput side directly in the direction of correction.

The adjustment is made by an assistant (or parent) with a gloved finger taking an intraoral contact on the maxilla on the side with the flat forehead and pulling laterally in the direction of correction of the strain (Figure 7.15). The doctor may need to request the pull to be slightly anterior or posterior as well as lateral until a release or 'give' has been felt.

If an underlying anterior–posterior strain is present, the infant's head will tend now to assume this pattern. This should be tackled on the next treatment a few days later, although both patterns can occasionally be corrected at the same visit.

Sphenobasilar torsion

A sphenobasilar torsion represents a twist at the sphenobasilar symphysis, the occiput being inferior on one side and the sphenoid superior on the same side. It is a common presentation

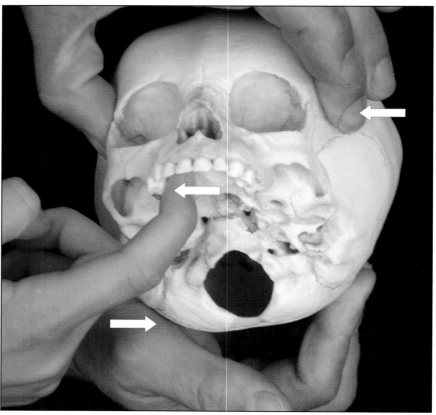
Figure 7.15 Correction of a lateral strain.

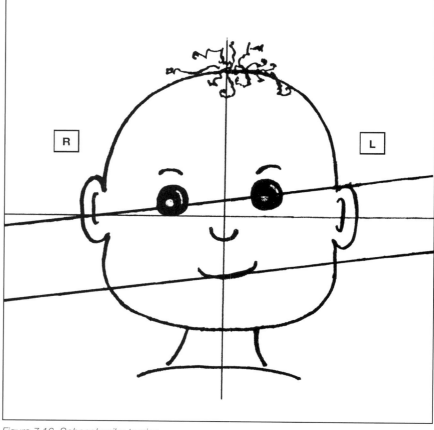
Figure 7.16 Sphenobasilar torsion.

and is recognised by the infant's eyes sloping down on one side in relation to his or her ears. The maxilla is level with the eyes in a torsion as there is no twist of the sphenomaxillary junction (Figure 7.16).

This strain is important to correct when the child is young: if it continues into later childhood and adulthood, people with it will tend to carry their head in slight lateral flexion to level their eyes to the floor. This then often leads to headaches and poor cervical biomechanics.

Correction

The doctor contacts the occiput and bridges over the frontal to contact the sphenoid bone, as in the correction of an anterior–posterior strain (see above). The doctor then induces a corrective torsion into the sphenobasilar symphysis by rotation of the occiput and sphenoid bones in opposite directions.

The adjustment is made by an assistant (or parent) inserting a gloved finger into the infant's mouth and contacting the infant's maxilla on the side of the low eye. A light pressure towards that eye is then used until a release is felt (Figure 7.17). The inter oral contact is essential to the correction.

Side-bend

A side-bend (fan face) is torsion of the sphenobasilar symphysis

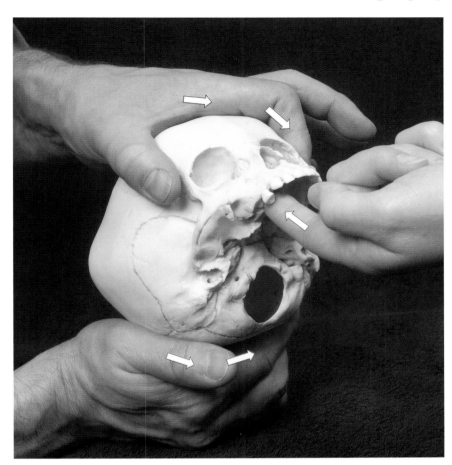

Figure 7.17 Correction of a sphenobasilar torsion.

with the addition of torsion of the sphenomaxillary junction in the opposite direction. In my experience, this is usually a cranial trauma pattern created either by forceps delivery or, in older children, by extraction orthodontics. Side-bend strains in children and adults often make up a large proportion of patients with chronic head and face pain (Walker 1996).

Visually, the pattern presents on facial examination with the eyes sloping to one side in relation to the ears and the maxilla sloping in the opposite direction to the eyes, creating a wide side (flexion pattern) of the face on one side

and a narrow face (extension pattern) on the opposite side (Figure 7.18). Older individuals with a side-bend will often tilt their head to one side when they swallow to level their maxilla to the ground (Walker 1996).

Correction

The correction is the same as that detailed for torsion correction apart from the intraoral contact. This time, instead of lifting the maxilla on the side of the low eye, the maxilla is contacted and lifted on the side with the high eye in order to close the open side of the 'fan' (Figure 7.19). For maximum efficacy, correction is should be undertaken when the

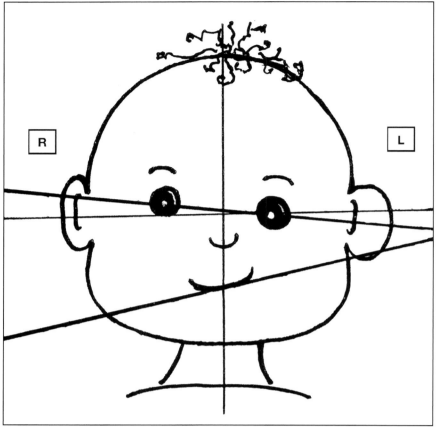

Figure 7.18 Left side-bend.

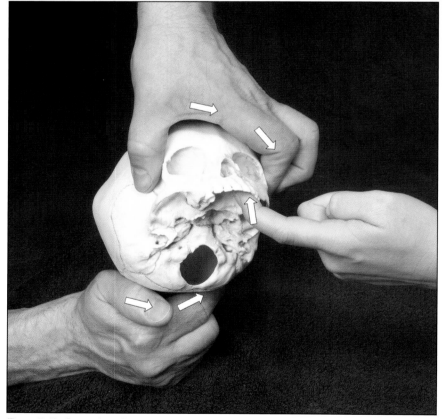

Figure 7.19 Correction of right side-bend.

child is as young as possible. It is, however, worth trying at any age as these individuals often suffer high levels of face and head pain that respond only in the short term to cervical adjusting.

Plate strain (unilateral posterior skull flattening)

Plate strains show a unilateral posterior skull flattening, usually over the occipitomastoid and lamboid suture areas (Figure 7.20). They are predisposed to by upper cervical rotary subluxations, which cause the infant to lie constantly on that area, leading to skull deformation. The anterior part of the skull is unaffected, differentiating the plate strain from an anterior–posterior strain. This strain pattern can be very resistant to correction, especially if the sleeping position cannot be altered. A device consisting of two triangular wedges to lay either side of the baby in order to control the sleeping position is very useful in this regard (available from smartazzkids.com).

Correction

Any upper cervical subluxation should be addressed prior to cranial correction, and in young infants this can, when combined with an alteration in sleeping position, be an effective treatment. In older infants (usually more than 3 months of age) cranial correction is also often needed. Farmer (2004) has developed a cranial adjustment for headache in adults, which also is useful in plate strain corrections in infants.

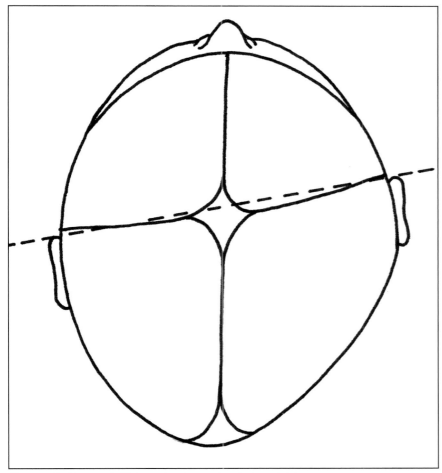

Figure 7.20 Plate strain (deformational posterior plagiocephaly).

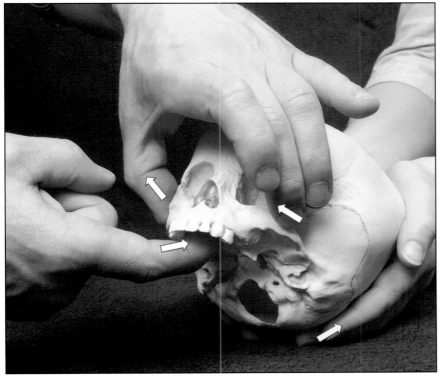

Figure 7.21 Correction of plate strain (deformational posterior plagiocephaly).

An assistant contacts the flattened area and tries, with the fingertips, gently to draw out the flattened occiput. The doctor contacts the zygomatic arches with a finger and a thumb bridging over the face and lifts superiorly (away from the face). The adjustment is made by doctor's gloved finger contacting the maxillopalatine suture on the side of flattening and lifting it towards the flat area of the skull (Figure 7.21). The doctor may need to alter his or her vectors slightly until a release is felt and the adjustment is complete. This adjustment needs to be repeated a number of times, and an alteration in the infant's sleeping position is essential to its success.

Case study

This case study describes baby James, who presented at 18 weeks old suffering from colic and plagiocephaly. He held his head in right rotation and did not like turning to the left. Delivery had been 3.5 hours from the start of contractions, and James was born with the cord round his neck. His parents commented that his head was initially fairly symmetrical.

On examination, his primitive reflex profile was unremarkable, and no neurological deficit was noted. Subluxations were noted at C1–C2 and T4–T5, and James' sacrum was posterior on the left. A diagnosis of a KISS 1 syndrome and deformational plagiocephaly was made. The skull strain, as can be seen from Figure 7.22, was a combination of lateral and anterior–posterior strains.

Treatment was initially focused on pelvic correction, and the anterior–posterior strain component was adjusted. At the third treatment, correction of the lateral strain component was undertaken. After four visits, there was a significant improvement in the cranial strain (Figure 7.23), and James is currently under maintenance care.

CONCLUSION

As with all the specific corrections I have detailed in this chapter, sacral and pelvic corrections, as described in Chapter 6, should be undertaken prior to the skull strain-specific corrections and are a prerequisite for a successful result and avoiding negative reactions to treatment. In older children, the release of jammed sutures is indicated prior to attempting strain correction as these sutures will otherwise tend to restrict the amount of correction that can be achieved.

It is of vital importance to the successful treatment of skull strains that the utmost gentleness and sensitivity be used in their correction .

Doctors attempting these corrections should be confident in their own ability in and experience of cranial work before using them. If correction does not occur, **DO NOT** use force; instead, try changing the vectors or revaluate the diagnosis.

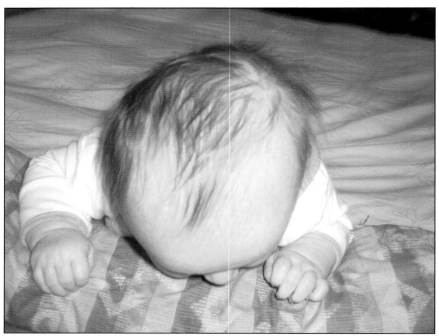

Figure 7.22 James – before correction of his lateral/anterior–posterior strain.

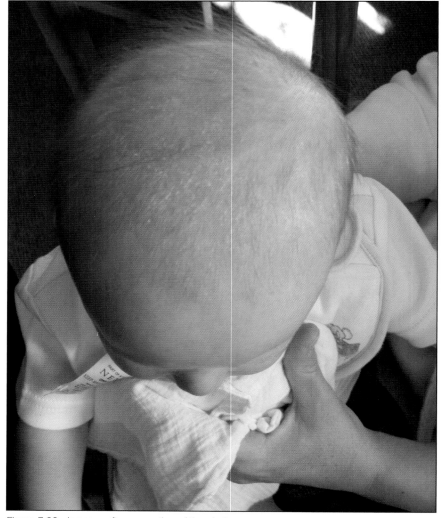

Figure 7.23 James – after correction of the strain.

REFERENCES

American Academy of Pediatrics. Prevention and management of positional skull deformities in infants. *Pediatrics* 2003; 112: 199–202.

Arbuckle BE. *The Selected Writings of Beryl E Arbuckle*. Indianapolis: American Academy of Osteopathy; 1994.

Biedermann H. Manual therapy in children: proposals for an etiologic model. *J Manipulative Physiol Ther* 2005; 28: e1.

Boere-Boonekamp MM, van der Linden-Kuiper LT. Positional preference: prevalence in infants and follow-up after two years. *Pediatrics* 2001; 107: 339–343.

Bruneteau RJ, Mulliken JB. Frontal plagiocephaly: synostotic, compensational, or deformational. *Plast Reconstr Surg* 1992; 89: 21–31; discussion 32–33.

Carreiro JE. *An Osteopathic Approach to Children*. Edinburgh: Churchill Livingstone, 2003.

Clarren SK. Plagiocephaly and torticollis, etiology, natural history and helmet treatment. *J Pediatr* 1981; 98: 92–95.

Davies NJ. Chiropractic management of deformational plagiocephaly. An alternative to device-dependant therapy. *Chiropr J Aust* 2002; 32: 52–55.

Farmer J. *Sacro occipital technique Seminar*. Omaha, Nebraska: Sacro Occipital Reasource International, October 2004.

Frymann V. The *Collected Papers of Viola M Frymann* DO. Indianapolis: American Academy of Osteopathy; 1998.

Glat PM, Freund RM, Spector JA, Levine J, Noz M, Bookstein FL, McCarthy JG, Cutting CB. A classification of plagiocephaly utilizing a three dimensional computer analysis of cranial base landmarks. *Ann Plast Surg* 1996; 36: 469–474.

Graham JM, Badura RJ, Smith DW. Coronal craniosynostosis: fetal head constraint as one possible cause. *Pediatrics* 1980; 65: 995–999.

Higginbottom MC, Jones KL, James HE. Intrauterine constraint and craniosynostosis. *Neurosurgery* 1980; 6: 39–44.

Kelly KM, Littlefield TR, Pomatto JK, Manwaring KH, Beals SP. Cranial growth unrestricted during treatment for deformational plagiocephaly. *Pediatr Neurosurg* 1999; 30: 193–199.

Kirschner RE, Gannon FH, Zu J, Wang J, Karmacharya J, Barlett SP, Whitaker LA. Craniosynostosis and altered patterns of fetal TGF-beta expression induced by intrauterine constraint. *Plast Reconstr Surg* 2002; 109: 2338–2346.

Little WJ. On the influence of abnormal parturition, difficult labour, premature birth and asphyxia neonatorum on the mental and physical conditions of the child especially in relation to deformities. *Trans Obstet Soc Lond* 1862; 3: 293–344.

Magoun HI. *Osteopathy in the Cranial Field*. Indianapolis: Academy of Osteopathy, 1976.

Miller RL, Clarren SK. Long term developmental outcomes in patients with deformational plagiocephaly. *Pediatrics* 2000; 105: e26.

Peitsch WK, Keefer CH, LaBrie RA, Mulliken JB. Incidence of cranial asymmetry in healthy newborns. *Pediatrics* 2002; 110: e72.

Upledger J, Vredevoogd JD. *Craniosacral Therapy*. Seattle: Eastland Press, 1983.

Walker RA. *Chirodontics seminar*. Oxford, UK, 1996.

Plagiocephaly

Illustrations in Chapter Seven

Chapter 8

Common paediatric syndromes amenable to chiropractic care and their management

This chapter is not meant to be a cookbook-style instruction manual on how to deal with specific problems, but merely an indication of where to look and focus care in each of the syndromes. When I began my paediatrics practice and was faced with crying babies with significant health issues, I felt I had few tools to assess them and was initially clueless on where to focus care. Very little had been written in chiropractic paediatrics at this time, and my undergraduate education in paediatrics was entirely medically orientated. This chapter is designed to take the stress off the chiropractor new to paediatrics and give technical aids to more experienced doctors. Each condition is looked at in terms of diagnosis, soft tissue releases, spinal treatment, cranial treatment, nutrition and supplementation.

COLIC

Infantile colic is one of the most common paediatric ills to present in the chiropractic office, thanks in part to some well-publicised Danish studies (Klougart et al 1989, Wiberg et al 1999) that showed a benefit from chiropractic care. In contrast, another study by Olafsdottir et al (2001) concluded that chiropractic was no more effective than placebo in the treatment of colic. However, their treatment methods (mobilisation techniques) were in my opinion not optimal, and they allowed only three sessions of chiropractic care in 8 days. A review of the recent studies involving chiropractic care for colic by Hughes and Bolton (2002), despite the somewhat ambivalent evidence, came out in favour of chiropractic care.

There are still arguments over exactly what colic entails, but a good depiction comes from Wessel et al (1954): "uncontrollable crying in an infant for more than 3 hours per day, often in the evening, for more than 3 days per week, for more than 3 weeks". Infants will often draw their legs up and gain relief from the passage of wind.

It seems likely that the lesion is a compression of the jugular foramen or torsion of the dura surrounding its contents, leading to irritation of the vagus nerve (Arbuckle 1994, Carriero 2003). The upper cervical spine is often involved owing to the distortion of the occipital condyles (the studies showing successful chiropractic interventions for colic focused on upper cervical adjustments). For a more complete and rapid response to care, it is, however, important in my experience also to take account of the soft tissue involvements.

Treatment

Soft tissue releases

Psoas and diaphragm (Figure 8.1) releases are particularly important, as diaphragm spasm seems to be one of the most common involvements in colic

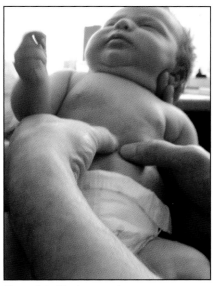

Figure 8.1 Diaphragm release.

105

Common paediatric syndromes

and indeed infant reflux. The adjustments are performed in the same way as described in the chapter on treatment of the pregnant female, but obviously on a smaller scale! Organ manipulation via chiropractic manipulative reflex technique, a development within Dejarnette's sacro occipital technique (Bathie 2000), is also useful, particularly the six-step correction for aiding gut mobility developed by Buddingh (1990).

The correction begins with the ileocaecal valve, located just below McBurney's point. This is held with light pressure or a gentle clockwise manipulation while the anterior head of the right humerus is manipulated until a release is felt under the fingers contacting over the ileocaecal valve (Figure 8.2a and 8.2b).

Then move half way up towards the rib cage on the right hand side of the abdomen to the ampulla of Vater (where the pancreatic duct joins the small intestine); this is held while manipulating the right radial head/extensor tendon area until relaxation or a gurgling is felt by the hand over the ampulla (Figure 8.3). The hand on the abdomen then contacts immediately under the right costal margin over the gallbladder, and the other hand manipulates the right thumb web. It can be helpful to traction the gallbladder toward the umbilicus until relaxation or a gurgle is felt (Figure 8.4).

Move on to the stomach reflex area 2.5 cm (1 inch) or so below the xiphoid process. Traction this inferiorly and manipulate the left thumb web until relaxation is felt (Figure 8.5a and 8.5b).

The pancreatic release is next, with a broad contact across the upper abdomen with one hand while manipulating the right thenar eminence with the other (Figure 8.6). The colon is then released with slow stretches applied to any area of excessive muscular tension – usually at the flexures – and fast stretches (slowly stretching the tissue and then releasing it with a fast separating stretch) are applied to any areas of flaccid muscular tone (Figure 8.7).

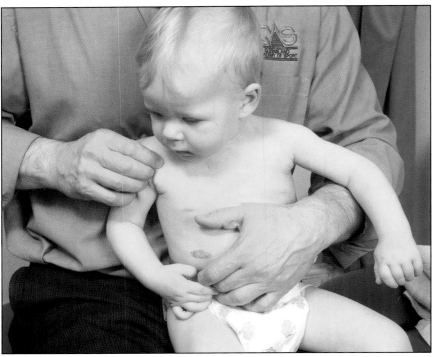

Figure 8.2a Ileocaecal valve release in the infant.

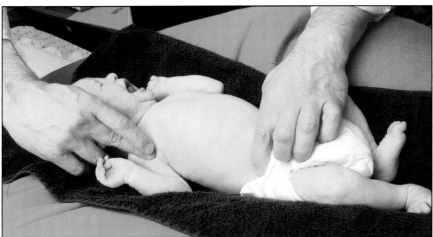

Figure 8.2b Ileocaecal valve release in the newborn.

106

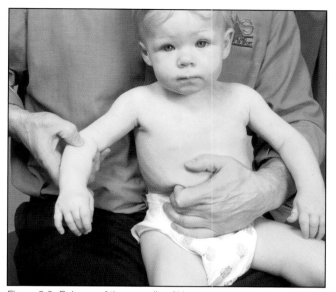

Figure 8.3 Release of the ampulla of Vater.

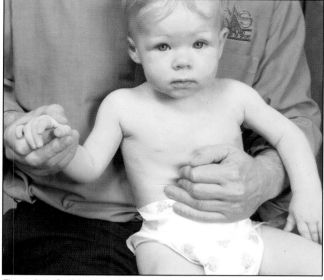

Figure 8.4 Gallbladder release.

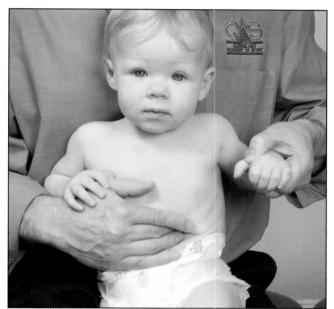

Figure 8.5a Stomach release.

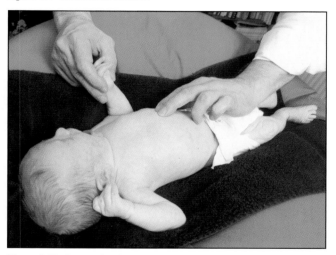

Figure 8.5b Stomach release in the newborn.

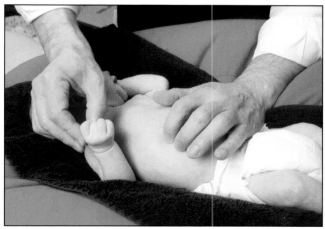

Figure 8.6 Pancreas release in the newborn.

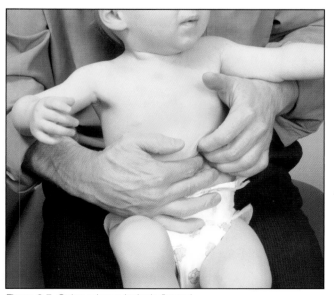

Figure 8.7 Colon release (splenic flexure).

Finish with a liver pump with one hand on the rib cage above the liver and one on the abdomen below, and gently compress the liver as if squeezing a sponge. This allows the blood in the liver to be replenished and to stimulate its activity (Figure 8.8).

This whole procedure takes about 3 minutes.

Spine

In colic, the levels of spinal involvement seem to be upper cervical vertebrae, C4–C5, T4–T5, the thoraco-lumbar junction and the sacrum (especially when constipation accompanies the colic).

Cranium

The primary cranial lesion present in colic appears to be an occipital compression, either unilateral or bilateral. Decompression of the occiput is indicated (Magoun 1976, Arbuckle 1994), as is balancing the sphenoid bone.

Diet

Sensitivity to formulae containing cow's milk derivatives is common in persistent colic (Lothe and Lindberg 1989), and a hypoallergenic formula should be sought. In older babies who are being weaned, the introduction of wheat and cow's milk products can create problems (it is best to wait until 1 year old when the interstitial spaces between the cells of the gut wall are tighter and more secure).

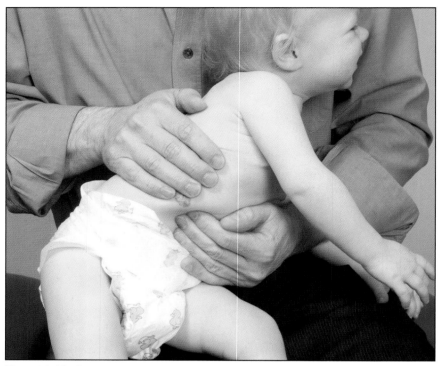

Figure 8.8 The liver pump.

Supplementation

I try to avoid supplementation in young babies, for the reason mentioned above.

FAILURE TO SUCKLE

Inability to suckle particularly on the breast is a common presentation and fortunately often a rewarding one to correct. If left untreated, however, it will often mean that mothers give up breast-feeding their infants and follow the easier road of bottle-feeding. Many mothers carry guilt into later life that they were unable to breast feed and are often initially referred to breast-feeding counsellors (lactation consultants). The fault is, however, all too often not with the mother's technique but with the baby's inability to suck properly.

Sucking can be first observed in utero as early as 18 weeks' gestation (Boyle 1992). However, premature infants of less than 32 weeks' gestation lack the ability to produce a coordinated and effective suck. Those born between 32 and 36 weeks do not have a mature sucking pattern, but it is somewhat more effective (Boyle 1992).

The nutritive suck (one that results in milk being released into the oral cavity) relies on a coordination of the tongue, hyoid, mandible and lower lip. This allows the tongue to be brought against the hard palate at a rapid rate (twice per second for 10–30 seconds), interspersed with between one and four swallows (Boyle 1992).

The oropharyngeal system is effectively suspended from the cranial base. The external muscles of the tongue attach to the mandible, temporal bone and hyoid. The hyoid is suspended from the temporal bones by the stylohyoid ligament and the stylohyoid and digastric muscles (Figure 8.9). The hyoid is attached to the sternum and clavicles by the sternohyoideus. From this, it can be seen that lesions of the clavicles and shoulder girdle, skull base and temporomandibular joint (TMJ) can interrupt effective sucking.

The nerve supply to the tongue is carried in the hypoglossal canal and exits at the hypoglossal foramen at the occipital condyle. The canal lies within the occipital condyle, which in neonates is cartilaginous in origin, and is in two parts (basilar and condylar portions), so the size and shape of the lumen may be compromised by distortions of these component parts (Carriero 2003). Several authorities (Magoun 1976, Arbuckle 1994) relate how weakened sucking activity occurs from irritation of the hypoglossal nerve at the level of the canal. True palsies will result in paresis of the ipsilateral muscles and a discordant tongue movement, with deviation towards the damaged side; fortunately, these are rare.

If the infant is unable to open his or her mouth wide because of TMJ dysfunction, the baby

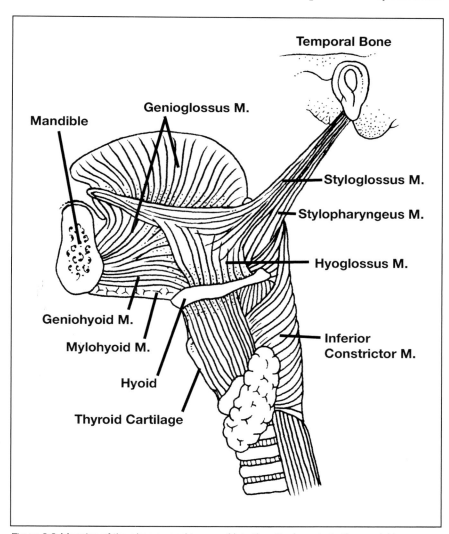

Figure 8.9 Muscles of the pharynx and tongue. Note the attachments to the cranial bones, hyoid and mandible. Adapted from Carreiro: An Osteopathic Approach to Children.

will not be able to cover the areolar area of the nipple, and dysfunctional feeding will result. These infants very often feed in short bursts and break off early, seeming to fatigue easily. Infants with compression or distortion of the maxilla often seem to exhibit an excessively strong suck and can create sore and cracked nipples for the mother. It may be that there is some effect on the proprioceptive feedback mechanisms of the infant that do not inform it that there is sufficient pressure as the infant sucks.

There is some evidence for musculoskeletal dysfunction and the effectiveness of manipulative treatment in infants with sucking disorders. Valone (2004), in a small comparative study of infants with breast-feeding difficulties, found an imbalanced musculoskeletal action compared with those who fed without a problem. Fraval (1998) found that osteopathic manipulation improved the effectiveness of sucking in infants with sucking disorders.

Treatment of sucking dysfunction

Soft tissue releases

First, release the muscles of the infant's throat. This is undertaken by holding the hyoid, with the infant supine and the neck in slight extension, the head then being gently rotated to one side until tension is felt. There will usually be a 'give' or a soft tissue release within a few seconds. The throat musculature is then released on the other side by rotating the head in the opposite direction. If no initial release is felt, try the opposite side and then return to the restricted side; this will then usually release easily (Figure 8.10a, 8.10b and 8.10c).

Any areas of restriction in the diaphragm should also be released – deviations in one transverse fascial plane of the baby cause deviations in others (diaphragm and thoracic outlet in this case). The muscles of the TMJ should be examined and released as necessary.

Spine

The upper cervical vertebrae should be checked and corrected, as should the upper thoracic vertebrae and anterior rib junctions.

Extremity

The glenohumeral, sterno-clavicular and acromio-clavicular joints should be checked and

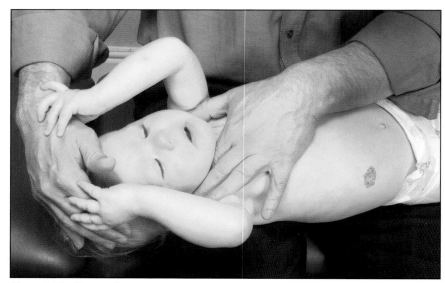
Figure 8.10a Throat release.

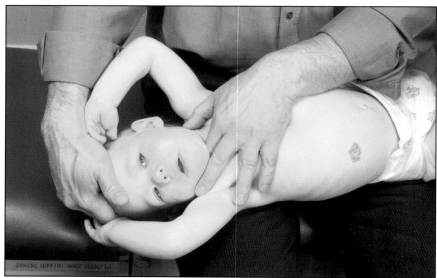
Figure 8.10b Throat release.

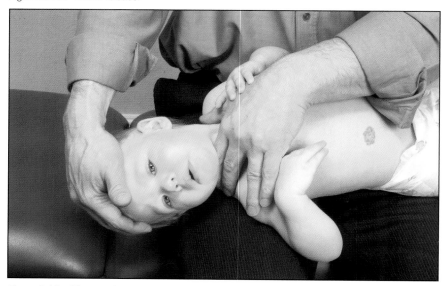
Figure 8.10c Throat release.

corrected if required (an activator is particularly useful in this regard).

The TMJ needs careful assessment. Subluxation of this joint is usually indicated by the infant's mouth deviating to one side on opening, which indicates an anterior displacement of the interosseous disc. The side of deviation is the side of disc displacement. Decompression of the joint is best accomplished from within the mouth, with the doctor's thumb on the mandibular ramus of the involved side. This is very gently pushed inferiorly and posteriorly until a release is felt and the disc is recaptured (Figure 8.11). This needs to be undertaken with the utmost sensitivity and care as the TMJ can be very vulnerable to damage and also very sensitive to pain.

Cranium

Cranial correction is the most important element in the treatment of sucking disorders. This is aimed at decompressing the component parts of the occiput, particularly the occipital condyles, and balancing the temporal bones (the ear-pull technique). Temporal bone balancing is important to the position and function of the TMJ as this bone houses the location of the mandibular condyle.

Diet

Breast-feeding is encouraged.

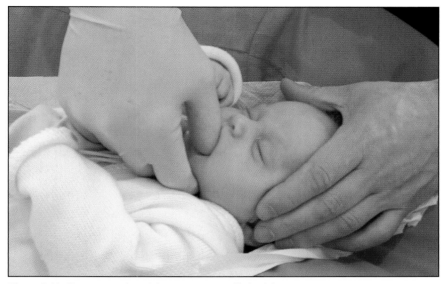

Figure 8.11 Decompression of the temporomandibular joint.

Supplementation

No supplementation is used at this time.

NOCTURNAL ENURESIS

Nocturnal enuresis (bed-wetting) is a complex problem, which can have a psychological involvement but often shows a beneficial response to chiropractic care.

Primary nocturnal enuresis is the most common type. This is defined as involuntary voiding of urine at night in a child 5 years or older who has never been continent for a prolonged period. At least one episode of bed-wetting per month occurs in 15–30% of 6-year-olds (a higher rate being seen in boys and children of Afro-Caribbean origin) and 4–16% of 12-year-olds (Sulkes and Dosa 2002). An organic aetiology is present in fewer than 1% of children with primary nocturnal enuresis.

Secondary nocturnal enuresis occurs when incontinence returns after a prolonged period of continence (3–6 months) and makes up about 20% of cases. It is usually the result of psychological stress (e.g. following parental separation) but does warrant investigation for an organic aetiology. A urinary tract infection is the most common organic cause, hence the need to dipstick the urine of all children you are considering for chiropractic care for blood, protein, glucose and white cells. Other less common organic causes include chemical urethritis from bubble bath, congenital anomalies, diabetes mellitus or insipidus and pelvic masses (including tumours and faecal impaction).

Primary nocturnal enuresis is deemed in the medical community to be due to a delay in the maturation of urethral sphincter control. Considering the success that chiropractic has in this condition, this may result from challenged neurological function. Distortions of the pubic symphysis often strongly affect bladder function; this may occur via the vesicular ligament, which attaches the pubis to the bladder.

The history is of prime importance when assessing a child for this condition because if there is a family history of late bladder control, especially involving the parents, this often means a poorer prognosis for the child in the short term (McMillan et al 1982).

As well as dipsticking the urine for the presence of white cells, blood, protein and glucose, it is also worthwhile measuring the volume of urine voided in 1 day. Forfar and Arneil (1973) have compiled a useful chart of urinary volumes (Table 8.1). If the child's age-related output is significantly above or below these levels, the child should be investigated for organic causes of nocturnal enuresis.

It is also worthwhile using a star chart for recording wet and dry nights for positive affirmation,

with agreed rewards being provided. This chart can also show patterns of wet nights, which can provide a clue to whether, for example, school stress is playing a part in the problem (Davies 2000). The bedding and/or nappies should be weighed each morning to check whether amounts of urine voided are decreasing with treatment.

Parental attitude is important: if the parents are also too fixated on the problem, this can stress the child and make the situation worse. Parents should be encouraged to try not to scold or blame the child as this can have the same effect.

Treatment of nocturnal enuresis

Soft tissues

Soft tissue corrections are in my experience very important to gain

balance in the urinary system. The areas commonly involved are the psoas muscles, kidneys, pelvic floor and vesicular ligament. Psoas release, kidney lift and pelvic floor balancing are all of vital importance in this condition and are covered in detail in Chapter 1.

The vesicular ligament is tested for excess tension by gently pressing a finger inferiorly behind the pubic bones on either side of the pubic symphysis (Barral 1993). The child lies supine with the knees bent and the feet flat on the table (Figure 8.12). The pressure is held until a subtle soft tissue give is felt. A feel for the correct degree of tension is gained only with practice. If the vesicular ligament is hypertonic, it can compromise bladder function, and a stretching release is indicated.

Chart of urinary volumes (Forfar and Arneil 1973)	
Age (years)	Volume (ml)
1–3	500–600 ml
3–4	600–700 ml
5–7	650–1000 ml
8–14	800–1400 ml

Table 8.1

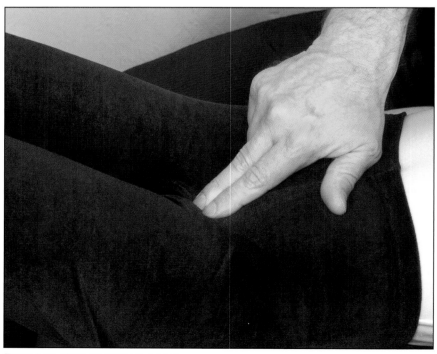

Figure 8.12 Vesicular ligament release.

Spine

The most important correction is that of a posterior S2 segment, which I usually adjust in side-posture as it needs a strong input into the adjustment to make a difference. Also worth checking are the lumbosacral and thoracolumbar junctions and, as with virtually all conditions, the upper cervical spine.

Cranium

The Lovett brother relationship (Lovett brother being a concept within applied kinesiology that involves the paired reciprocity of skeletal structures) for the sacrum is the occiput so this should be examined for good mobility.

Extremity

In my experience, femoral rotations are commonly involved in genitourinary problems. Probably because of the attachment of the obturator muscles to the femur and their relationship to the pelvic floor, so it is useful to check and correct the hip joints. I also regularly find an involvement of the pubic symphysis, particularly in girls. Assessment and correction of the pubic symphysis are covered in detail in Chapter 1.

Diet

Certain drinks, for example blackcurrant squash, juice or soda, and fizzy drinks, should be avoided as they tend to make the situation worse. Other foods and drinks can be tested using applied kinesiology to ascertain whether they are creating a problem.

A vital aspect, however, is not to reduce the fluid intake in the evening: it seems that the more concentrated the urine, the greater the irritation to the bladder and the more likely the child is to void urine while sleeping. Keeping hydrated by drinking plenty of water during the day is very important.

Supplementation

I have not found any specific supplementation to be useful for this condition, but I tend to advise parents to put their children on extra omega-3 oils and a broad-spectrum vitamin/mineral supplement, owing to common deficiencies in most children's diet.

OTITIS MEDIA

By 1 year of age, 50% of children will have had at least one episode of otitis media, and by 3 years of age this reaches over 70%. Up to one third of children will have six or more episodes before starting school, and some can have up to 12 episodes per year (Kline 1990). Signs and symptoms include pain, fever, vomiting, irritability, tugging at the ear and hearing loss. In some instances, otitis media may be asymptomatic and picked up only on routine otoscopic examination, when a fluid level or bulging of the tympanic membrane is noted. A colour change of the tympanic membrane is not a reliable indicator of infection in babies: it can flush simply because the baby is crying (Goldbloom 2003).

Risk factors include birth trauma (forceps, vacuum extraction and prolonged labour), low socio-economic status, the early introduction of solids, allergy, respiratory infection and poor nutritional status. There are high rates of otitis media in Down's syndrome and fetal alcohol syndrome (Schmidt 1996).

Medical treatments include antibiotics, antihistamines, decongestants and, in chronic cases, surgery. There is little evidence for the effectiveness of these therapies, and in the UK general practitioners are advised initially to prescribe only analgesia in cases of simple otitis media as the condition tends to be self-limiting (National Health Service 2003).

There is some indicative evidence for the effectiveness of chiropractic care, but as yet no randomised controlled trials have been carried out. Fysh (1996) presents a case series involving five children treated with chiropractic care who showed an excellent outcome. Froehle (1996), in a retrospective study of 46 children under the age of 5 years with an ear infection, demonstrated an improvement rate of 93% of all episodes, 75% occurring in 10 days or less. Fallon and Edelmen (1998) reported some encouraging results using chiropractic care in a pilot study of 401 children with otitis media. Tympanography was used as an objective measure.

Treatment of Otis Media

Soft tissues

Frymann (1998, p 110) stated that 'efficient lymphatic and venous drainage from the ear is dependent on anatomic-physiologic integrity of the jugular foramen and the cervical spine with its various fascial planes, of the superior thoracic outlet, the clavico-pectoral fascia and of the thoracic diaphragm'. Mechanical drainage of the regional lymphatic chains is indicated. This involves gentle stroking movements towards the base of the neck of the anterior and posterior auricular, submandibular, anterior and posterior cervical chains and the subclavicular lymph nodes.

Techniques aimed at draining the throat and opening up the fossa of Rosenmüller (the entrance into the pharynx of the eustachian tube) should be applied. The throat release described in the treatment for sucking dysfunction (Figure 8.10 above) is also useful in the treatment of

otitis media. Older children can help by moving their jaw as far as they can from side to side on a regular basis at home. This helps to open the eustachian tube, encourages drainage and may well have an effect on the tensor veli palatini, the muscle that opens the tube and is innervated by the mandibular branch of the trigeminal nerve.

A much more unpleasant technique can be helpful in older children and adults with recurrent otitis media. A gloved finger is passed behind the palatine tonsil and 'swept' laterally over the entrance to the eustachian tube, often with an osseous sounding release. When the eustachian tube is solidly blocked with mucous, this can have great results. Caution should, however, be exercised: it is unpleasant for the child, causing tearing and gagging, and bloody mucous is often left on the gloved finger. The procedure requires confidence on the part of the chiropractor, as well as the patient's full cooperation.

It is also useful to release the transverse facial planes of the respiratory diaphragm and the pelvic floor.

Spine

Adjustments to the upper cervical vertebrae, in particular C2 owing to its involvement with innervating the sternocleidomastoid muscle, are often required,

especially in acute otitis media. The upper thoracic spine and sacrum should also be carefully examined and corrected.

Cranium

The most important release is temporal decompression, which, when the child is under 3 years of age, is most easily accomplished using the ear-pull technique. In older children, the reciprocating temporal rocker technique is also useful (Chapter 6) to allow good temporal function. In addition, it is important to check and correct as required the zygomatic arches, sphenoid bones and occiput.

Temporomandibular joint

TMJ dysfunction can aggravate conditions involving ear drainage because of the proximity of the ear canal and the TMJ. Children who brux (grind their teeth) at night often are among the more stubborn cases to treat, especially if they have worn down their dentition to such an extent that they are severely overclosing and compressing the TMJ. Some cases necessitate the use of molar build-ups (Loudon 1990) or, in older children, dental splints to regain the necessary vertical height within the bite.

Decompression of the TMJ, as described for the treatment of sucking disorders, can be helpful, with the addition of trigger point work on the lateral pterygoid muscle.

Diet

Early cow's milk consumption may predispose to otitis media, and cow's milk is one of the most significant contributions to middle ear problems in children (Saarinen et al 1983). It may be difficult to avoid cow's milk for formula-fed babies, but there are formulae available that are hypoallergenic or based on goat's milk. Other foods that thicken the mucous are worth avoiding, at least initially, in acute or chronic disease. These include orange juice, peanuts and peanut butter, bananas, wheat, sugar and additives.

Feeding position is also very important. In a study of 2500 infants, the practice of giving a child a bottle in bed was the most important factor associated with persistent fluid in middle ear (Teele et al 1980). This may well be due in part to the horizontal position of the eustachian tube and the ease with which the fluid backs up into the tube. Niemela et al (2000) found similar problems with the use of a dummy (pacifier), which they suggested might be due to pressure changes in the nasopharynx and subsequent impaired function of the eustachian tube.

Supplements

Zinc deficiency has been linked both to generalised reduced immunity (Golden et al 1977) and, specifically, to otitis media (Bondestam et al 1985). Other useful supplements include vitamins A and C. I generally avoid recommending supplementation for a child under 1 year of age, apart from probiotics when infants have been given antibiotics.

The dosage must reflect the size of the individual: if the dosage of zinc given to an adult were 30–50 mg and the child were one quarter of adult size, the dosage would be 5–10 mg per day. Essential fatty acids are also very important in producing anti-inflammatory prostaglandins; they are also very commonly deficient in the modern diet.

Recommendations for daily intake are given in Table 8.2.

ASTHMA

Asthma is defined as the reversible obstruction of large and small airways as the result of a hyperresponsiveness to various immunological and non-immunological stimuli (Tepas and Umetsu 2002).

Diagnosis

The disease is characterised by recurrent episodes of cough, chest tightness, dyspnoea and wheezing. In the USA, 5 million children have asthma, and that figure is expected to double by 2020 (Tepas and Umetsu 2002).

The causes are not well understood but appear to be multifactorial. Vaccination (especially against pertussis) has been blamed in some alternative medicine circles but with little hard evidence. Pollution and a decreased exposure to bacteria and dirt with the modern emphasis on cleanliness and the decrease in airflow in Western houses has also recently come into focus. Whatever the reason, the condition is certainly becoming much more common.

Many chiropractors have experienced beneficial effects for their patients from chiropractic spinal adjusting, without much solid research backing this up. My contention is that spinal adjusting alone is not enough and attention needs to be paid to the whole mechanics of the respiratory system, from the cranium to the diaphragm and viscera, and not just to spinal joints.

Recommendations for daily intake in otitis media (Schmidt 1996)		
	Age 1-3 years	Age 4 and above
Vitamin C	500 mg (powder)	1.0–1.5 mg
Beta-carotene	5000 IU	5000 IU
Zinc	5–10 mg	10 mg
Flaxseed oil	5 ml	7.5 ml
Star flower oil	2.5 ml	5 ml

Table 8.2

Evidence

Balon et al (1998) reported an interesting study that showed no statistical difference between the group receiving chiropractic treatment (thoracic manipulation) and the control group. It should be noted, however, that the control group received a 'sham' treatment composed of techniques quite similar to osteopathic soft tissue techniques. An osteopathic study by Fitzgerald and Styles (1984) reported a 14% decrease in the length of hospital stay when osteopathic manipulation was added to the management of adult patients with asthma.

A number of case reports in the literature describe the efficiency of chiropractic care for asthmatic children (Arbiloff 1969, Mega 1982, Cohen 1988, Garde 1994, Burnier 1995); although useful as indicators for further study, these results alone are not solid evidence of the benefit of chiropractic care. Two randomised clinical trails of chiropractic spinal manipulative therapy (Nielson et al 1995, Bronfort et al 2001) showed no significant objective improvement in lung function. Both, however, showed the subjective ratings of their asthma by patients to be significantly improved.

Treatment of Asthma

Soft tissue

Release of the psoas muscles and diaphragm are important for lung function generally. If the diaphragm is restricted, the child will not be able to use the lower third of his or her lungs effectively. Diaphragm release is best performed using the methods out lined in Chapter 1, some accommodation being made for the fact that children often find these procedures ticklish – although this makes the treatment fun!

Release of the sternocostal and costochondral junctions is also very effective in increasing lung function in asthmatics. Patients with uncontrolled asthma can become barrel-chested, and even in well-controlled chronic asthma, these junctions become tight, decreasing the efficiency of lung function. One of the easiest and least uncomfortable methods of correction for the anterior rib junctions uses a racket ball to torque the cartilaginous junction into the direction of greatest restriction and release it with a fast twist (Figure 8.13). This can be then applied to all the anterior rib junctions in turn.

Barral (2001), in his book on manipulation of the thorax, describes a technique to balance the fascia of the lungs and lung lobes. I find this technique clinically very useful, and it often results in the patient being

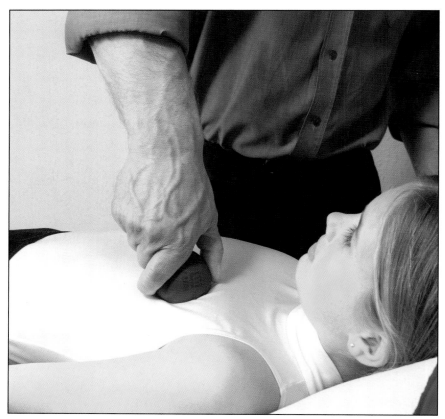

Figure 8.13 Costochondral release.

able to shift a mucous build-up more easily. This technique involves placing full-hand contact over adjacent lung lobes on the same side and feeling for the movement of the individual lobes during normal breathing. A significant difference will often be noted, with one moving well and the other being less mobile.

The less mobile lobe needs to be induced into movement so a fascial release is performed, taking it in the direction of freedom or easiest movement. This often involves a twist or lateral or medial shift. Follow this fascial release until movement of the lung lobes becomes balanced (Figure 8.14). This involves only one application on the left because two lobes are present, but it obviously needs to be done twice on the right owing to the additional lobe.

Visceral manipulation of the gallbladder surprisingly often seems to be effective in helping young asthmatics, but the underlying mechanism is unclear.

Extremity

It is very important that the clavicles are freely mobile as they facilitate full expansion of the upper part of the lungs and chest wall. In chronic asthma, the accessory muscles of respiration often become tight, and the sternocleidomastoid and scalene muscles pull on and lock the upper ribs and clavicles.

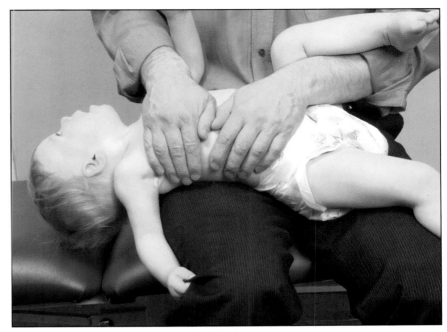

Figure 8.14 Balancing the lung lobes – fascial release.

The clavicles are most effectively freed up by placing the child supine and hooking under the superior aspect of the clavicle with one hand. The other hand holds the ipsilateral arm of the patient out at 90 degrees and rotates it in large circles while trying to work the fingers under the clavicle. The adjustment is finished with the patient's arm vertical and pulled towards the ceiling while the doctor's fingers under the clavicle try to lift it ceiling-wards off the ribs (Figure 8.15). This should be undertaken with care as it can be quite uncomfortable.

Spine

The upper cervical vertebrae should be checked and corrected as necessary, as should C4–C5 because of the phrenic nerve. Upper and mid-thoracic subluxations, usually around T3–

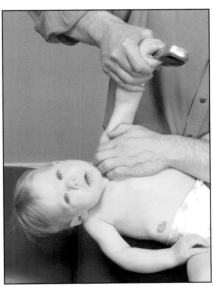

Figure 8.15 Clavicle release and lift.

T4, seem to be very common, and it is also worth checking the thoracolumbar junction and the second sacral area.

Cranium

Occipital decompression is essential, especially among younger asthmatics, because any compression of the jugular foramen or dural tension in this area can irritate the vagus, which is part of the parasympathetic supply to the lungs.

Another technique, which can prove effective in decompressing the jugular foramen, is Buddingh and Skiptead's (2003) jugular foramen decompression. The indicators for this technique are the weakening of a strong indicator muscle on head and body lateral flexion (Figure 8.16a) – indicating a lesion on the side of lateral flexion – and the weakening of a strong indicator muscle on foot plantarflexion (Figure 8.16b), opposite to the side of the lesion.

Correction is achieved by inserting a gloved finger into the mouth and hooking behind the alveolar bone of the maxilla on the side being adjusted with that finger. The external hand contacts the temporal bone behind the ear, and the internal finger pulls gently away from the temporal bone, attempting to 'separate' the two and open up the jugular foramen (Figure 8.17). If a child is old enough, ask him or her to breathe in and out deeply two or three times to facilitate this separation.

Dejarnette (1979) mentions that the temporal bones are often involved in repetitive coughs. The first sign of asthma in babies is often a repetitive night cough, and coughing in asthma certainly contributes to closing of the airways. Clinically, I have found that balancing the temporal bones using the ear-pull technique is

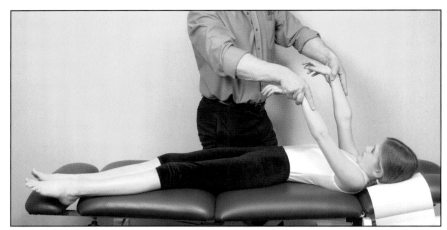

Figure 8.16a Jugular foramen compression test: lateral flexion.

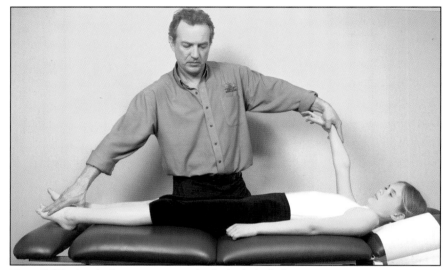

Figure 8.16b Jugular foramen compression test: plantarflexion.

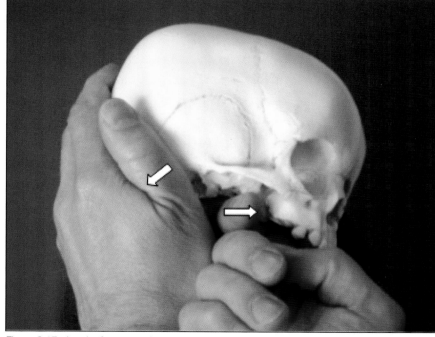

Figure 8.17 Jugular foramen release.

useful in controlling asthma in children with tickly, recurrent coughs. This is probably because of the temporal bone's connection to the eustachian tube and its opening in the throat, mucous discharge from it causing throat irritation and coughing.

There are several techniques taught within sacro occipital technique that are 'specific' for asthma and useful in older children. These include cruciate suture technique and sphenobasilar-occipito-frontal technique; for these, refer to the cranial specifics section of the sacro occipital technique cranial participant guide (Saxon and Decamp 1990).

Diet

The consumption of oily fish has been linked to a significantly reduced risk of asthma (Hodge et al 1996).

The avoidance of additives and colourings is important in some forms of asthma and, as a ground rule, all should be avoided. Surrogate testing or direct kinesiologic testing of the child can be performed to ascertain whether any food types are causing sensitivities. The foods that most commonly produce a reaction in asthma are, in my experience, dairy products, wheat, juices (particularly orange) and refined sugar.

Supplementation

Supplements of pycnogenol (a bioflavonoid from the French maritime pine) significantly improved lung function in a small randomised controlled trial (60 subjects) of childhood asthmatics (Lau et al 2004).

Increased serum levels of antioxidants (selenium, vitamin C, vitamin E and beta-carotene) are associated with a reduction (of up to 50%) in the prevalence of asthma in children (Rubin et al 2004). If the asthmatic child will not eat oily fish and a high antioxidant-based diet, supplementation would appear to be indicated.

If the immune system appears to be compromised with recurrent respiratory infections, supplementation with vitamin A to a maximum of 5000 IU per day can be useful. Higher doses of beta-carotene are acceptable, as are vitamin C (powered and buffered to bowel tolerance), zinc (up to 20 mg per day) and omega-3 oils. A protocol similar to that detailed by Schmidt (1996) in the section on otitis media may be followed.

CEREBRAL PALSY

Cerebral palsy includes a variety of non-degenerating neurological disabilities caused by abnormal central nervous system development, as well as injuries in the prenatal, perinatal and early postpartum period causing abnormalities of motor function (Sulkes and Dosa 2002). The incidence is about 2.5 per 1000 live births.

Birth anoxia is probably the most common cause – 25% of cases in one large study (Laisram et al 1992). Risk factors include maternal hormone treatment, low socio-economic status, maternal seizures, polyhydramnios, eclampsia, third-trimester bleeding, twin pregnancy, fetal growth retardation, abnormal presentation and premature separation of the placenta (Kuban and Levinton 1994). Apgar scores of 3 or less at 20 minutes are associated with a 250-fold increase in the risk of cerebral palsy (Roosenbloom 1995).

Classification can be made by physiological type or distribution. When classified by physiological type, spastic cerebral palsy is the most common, occurring in 70–80% of individuals. Dyskinetic cerebral palsy occurs in about 10–15% of individuals with cerebral palsy. Ataxic cerebral palsy makes up fewer than 5% of cases, and mixed cerebral palsy 10–15% of cases (Sulkes and Dosa 2002). My experience has been mainly with spastic and mixed cerebral palsy, and the following treatment strategies are generally primarily for helping children with spasticity and balance problems.

Spastic cerebral palsy often presents with a limited regional distribution. Spastic diplegia, for example, involves the lower extremities, occurs in 25–35% of cases and is often related to low birthweight (Sulkes and Dosa 2002). Spastic quadriplegia involves all four limbs, is found in 40–50% of cases and is associated with greater neurological and orthopaedic consequences. Spastic hemiplegia involves 25–40% of cases.

Approximately one third of children with cerebral palsy have epilepsy, and 30–70% show significant cognitive impairments (Sulkes and Dosa 2002).

There are a number of case reports in the chiropractic literature of improvements, some very marked, following chiropractic care (Sweat and Ammons 1988, Golden and Van Egmond 1992, Collins 1994, Webster 1994, McCoy et al 2000). There is also some strong evidence from the related field of manual medicine for the use of manipulation and fascial release techniques in cerebral palsy (Lohse-Busch 2003, Lohse-Busch et al 2003).

Treatment of Cerebral Palsy

Soft tissues

There are many soft tissue distortion patterns present in cases of cerebral palsy, and great attention needs to be paid to them. Transverse fascial plane balancing involving the psoas, diaphragm (Figure 8.18) and pelvic floor is a good first step.

The contractions that occur in the limbs need stretching (Figure 8.19), which in most cases the

parents or carers do at home. This is particularly important for the lower limb muscles in order to allow the possibility of walking. Numerous stretching and neuromuscular techniques can be employed with good effect. I favour active release technique as, in my experience, it allows muscle fascial adhesions to be broken down progressively.

Treatment should begin at as young an age as possible in order to avoid bony distortions permanently affecting the pelvis. Carreiro (2003) stresses the importance of lower limb muscle function in terms of the femoral-acetabular relationship. She states that chronic muscle spasm of the biceps femoris will increase inferior tension on the ischial

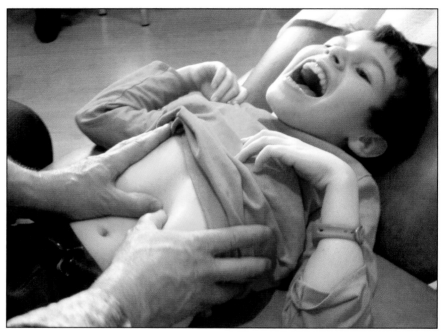

Figure 8.18 Diaphragm release.

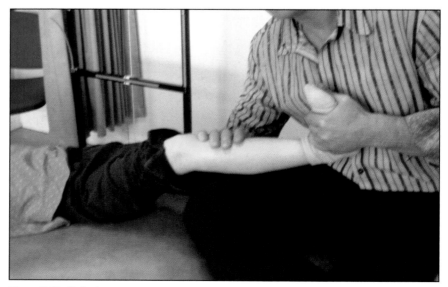

Figure 8.19 Calf release.

120

component of the acetabulum (as the pubic bone, ischium and ileum join at the centre of the acetabulum), affecting the shape of the acetabular space and compromising the relationship of the joint. Children who have hypertonicity of the lower extremities will have altered hip relations because of their relatively flat acetabulum, which may lead to distortion or a slipped capital femoral epiphysis (Carreiro 2003).

Increased tone in the hamstrings in spastic hemiplegic or diplegic cerebral palsy will tend to cause posterior rotation of the ipsilateral innominate bone, resulting in a loss of the lumbar lordosis. If the child is upright, he or she will compensate by extending at the thoracolumbar junction, which leads to flattening of the normal thoracic kyphosis extending the occiput on the atlas. This may shift the centre of gravity in an anterior–superior direction, altering respiratory mechanisms and causing compression of the cranial bones. These children will also tend to sit in a slumped posture because increased hamstring tone rotates the innominate bones posteriorly and tips the pelvis backwards.

Muscle-stretching techniques for the extremities are indicated in younger children, but as they get older and are able to follow instructions, techniques such as osteopathic muscle energy techniques, strain–counterstrain and proprioceptive neuromuscular facilitation are also effective. Indirect fascial release techniques are very useful in 'unwinding' many of the restrictions caused by the chronic muscle tension and should be used as part of the treatment programme.

Extremity

Extremity adjusting is of the utmost importance to children with cerebral palsy in order to improve function and decrease joint pain, which often occurs as they try to use their limbs against the muscle contractions.

Toe-walking as a result of extreme tension is usually treated with a rigid orthotic device that holds the ankle joint into dorsiflexion. Unfortunately, these very often tend to drive to foot into eversion, causing more strain on the plantar arch. This in turn tends to rotate the tibia medially and cause the navicular to fall inwards. Adjustments are needed to the calcaneus, navicular, cuboid and the tarsal bones; this will often regain some plasticity in the arch (Figure 8.20). If the pes planus caused by the rigid orthotic is not dealt with, the medial tibia rotation can result in a permanent twist within the tibia.

It is important therefore to attempt to enable a cerebral palsy child to cope without rigid orthotics (obviously with the co-operation of other professionals involved in their care) if at all possible, although a foot orthosis that attempts to put the rear foot in neutral is usually helpful.

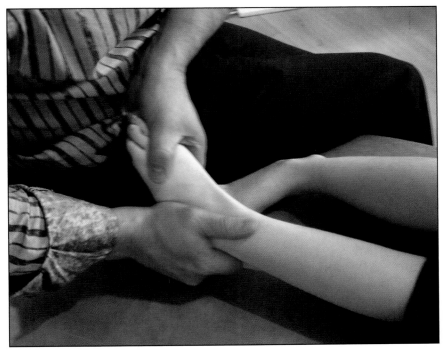

Figure 8.20 Cuboid adjustment.

Regular adjustments of the feet ankles and knees are indicated. In severe cases, however, it may be necessary to refer for temporary lower limb casts, which progressively stretch in particular the Achilles tendons, or even for the surgical correction of resistant cases.

Spine

The upper cervical spine should be assessed thoroughly and treated if necessary. McMullen (1990) commented that, in her experience of treating cerebral palsy, the occipito-atlantal articulation was the area most commonly subluxated.

The thoracic spine and rib cage also require close attention, as does the pelvis because the postural patterns derived by the chronically tight muscles will tend to cause recurrent subluxation patterns in these areas. Arbuckle (1994) recommends that, after cranial correction, the upper thoracic spine is manipulated to improve cranial circulation by stimulating the autonomic nervous system.

Cranium

Cranial restriction patterns, particularly involving the cranial base, are extremely common in cerebral palsy. Arbuckle (1994) found that many babies exhibiting signs of spasticity had a rotation of the occipital squama with compensatory flattening of the opposite parietal bone. She further stated that early treatment of this cranial pattern could minimise the spasticity. I have found this pattern to be common in children with spastic cerebral palsy.

In cerebral palsy, the whole cranium needs attention, but specific corrections involving occipital, temporal and frontal decompression are of particular use. If there is significant spasticity in the lower extremities, it is very helpful to have an assistant (or parent) to straighten the legs and dorsiflex the child's feet during the cranial releases. There is so much fascial tension in cerebral palsy that it is useful to have an anchor point from which to release the cranium.

Diet

If food sensitivities are suspected, they should be tested for and avoided.

Supplementation

Because of the difficulties some children with cerebral palsy have with chewing and swallowing, a general multivitamin/mineral and additional fatty acid supplement are indicated. These may, however, have to be in liquid form and mixed with food or drink if the child cannot swallow capsules or tablets.

REFERENCES

Colic

Arbuckle BE. *The Collected Writings of Beryl E Arbuckle.* Indianapolis: American Academy of Osteopathy, 1994.

Bathie R. *Chiropractic Manipulative Reflex Technique Manual.* Prairie Village, Kansas: Sacro Occipital Resource International, 2000.

Buddingh K. *Occipital Fiber Nutrition.* Private publication, Los Angeles, 1990.

Carreiro JE. *An Osteopathic Approach to Children.* Edinburgh: Churchill Livingstone, 2003.

Hughes S, Bolton J. Is chiropractic an effective treatment of infantile colic? *Arch Dis Child* 2002; 86: 382–384.

Klougart N, Nilsson N, Jacobsen J. Infantile colic treated by chiropractors: a prospective study of 316 cases. *J Manipulative Physiol Ther* 1989; 12: 281–288.

Lothe L, Lindberg T. Cows milk whey protein elicits symptoms of infantile colic in colicky formula fed infants: a double blind crossover study. *Pediatrics* 1989; 83: 262–266.

Magoun HI. *Osteopathy in the Cranial Field.* Indianapolis: Cranial Academy, 1976.

Olafsdottir E, Forshei S, Fluge G, Markestad T. Randomised controlled trial of infantile colic treated with chiropractic spinal manipulation. *Arch Dis Child* 2001; 84: 138–141.

Wessel MA, Cobb JC, Jackson ES, Harris GS, Detwiler AC. Paroxysmal fussing in infancy sometimes called colic. *Pediatrics* 1954; 14: 421–434.

Wiberg JMM, Nordsteen J, Nilsson N. The short term effect of spinal manipulation in the treatment of infantile colic: a randomized controlled trial with a blinded observer. *J Manipulative Physiol Ther* 1999; 22: 517–522.

Failure to suckle

Arbuckle BE. *The Collected Writings of Beryl E Arbuckle.* Indianapolis: American Academy of Osteopathy, 1994.

Boyle J. Motility of the upper gastrointestinal tact in the fetus and neonate. In *Fetal and Neonatal Physiology*, Pollin R, Fox W (eds). Philadelphia: WB Saunders, 1992.

Carreiro JE. *An Osteopathic Approach to Children.* Edinburgh: Churchill Livingstone, 2003.

Fraval M. A pilot study: osteopathic treatment of infants with sucking dysfunction. *Am Acc Osteopathy J* 1998; Summer: 25–33.

Magoun HI. *Osteopathy in the Cranial Field.* Indianapolis: Cranial Academy, 1976.

Valone S. Chiropractic evaluation and treatment of musculoskeletal dysfunction in infants demonstrating difficulty breast feeding. *J Clinical Chiro Pediatr* 2004; 6: 349–366.

Nocturnal enuresis

Barral J-P. *Urogenital Manipulation.* Washington: Eastland Press, 1993.

Davies NJ. The enuretic child. *In Chiropractic Paediatrics*, Davies NJ (ed.). Edinburgh: Churchill Livingstone, 2000, pp 187–195.

Forfar J, Arneil G. *Textbook of Pediatrics.* Edinburgh: Churchill Livingstone, 1973.

McMillan JA, Stockman JA, Oski FA. *The Whole Pediatrician Catalogue.* Philadelphia: WB Saunders, 1982.

Sulkes SB, Dosa NP. Developmental and behavioral pediatrics. In *Nelson's Essentials of Pediatrics, 4th edn*, Berhman RE, Kliegman RM (eds). Philadelphia: WB Saunders, 2002, pp 1–56.

Otitis media

Bondestam M, Foccard T, Gebre-Medhin M. Subclinical trace element deficiency in children with undue susceptibility to infections. *Acta Paediatr Scand* 1985; 74: 515–520.

Fallon J, Edelman MJ. Chiropractic care of 401 children with otitis media: a pilot study. *Altern Ther Health Med* 1998; 4: 93.

Froehle RM. Ear infection: a retrospective study examining improvement from chiropractic care and analyzing for influencing factors. *J Manipulative Physiol Ther* 1996; 19: 196–177.

Frymann VM. Diagnosis and treatment of otitis media in children. In *The Collected Papers of Viola M Frymann DO*. Indianapolis: American Academy of Osteopathy, 1988.

Fysh PN. Chronic recurrent otitis media: case series of five patients with recommendations for management. *J Clin Chiropr Pediatr* 1996; 1: 66–77.

Goldbloom RB. *Pediatric Clinical Skills, 3rd edn*. Philadelphia: WB Saunders, 2003.

Golden M, Jackson A, Golden B. Effect of zinc on the thymus of recently malnourished children. *Lancet* 1977; ii: 1057–1059.

Kline MW. Otitis media. In *Principles and Practice of Pediatrics*, Oski FA, DeAngelis CD, Feigin RD, Warshaw JB (eds). Philadelphia: JB Lippincott, 1990.

Loudon ME. Recent advancements in vertical dimension: primary molar buildups. *Funct Orthod* 1990; 7: 10–17.

National Health Service. Diagnosis and Management of Childhood Otitis Media in Primary Care. *NHS*, 2003.

Niemela M, Pihakari O, Pokka T, Uhari M. Pacifier as a risk factor for acute otitis media: a randomized controlled trial of parental counseling. *Pediatrics* 2000; 106: 483–488.

Saarinen U, Savilahti E, Arjomaa P. Increased IgM-type betalactoglobulin antibodies in children with recurrent otitis media. *Allergy* 1983; 38: 571–576.

Schmidt M. *Healing Childhood Ear Infections*. Berkley, California: North Atlantic Books, 1996.

Teele DW, Klein JO, Rosner BA. Epidemiology of otitis media in children. *Ann Otol Rhinol Laryngol* 1980; 89 (pt 3 suppl 68): 5–6.

Asthma

Arbiloff B. Bronchial asthma: a case report. *J Clin Chiropr* 1969; 2: 40–42.

Balon J, Aker PD, Crowther ER., Danielson C, Cox PG, O'Shaughnessy D, Walker C, Goldsmith CH, Duku E, Sears MR. A comparison of active and simulated chiropractic manipulation as an adjunctive treatment for childhood asthma. *N Engl J Med* 1998; 339: 1013–1020.

Barral J-P. *The Thorax*. Seattle: Eastland Press, 2001.

Brontfort G, Evans RL, Kubic P, Filkin P. Chronic pediatric asthma and chiropractic manipulation; a prospective clinical series and randomized pilot study. *J Manipulative Physiol Ther* 2001; 24: 369–377.

Buddingh K, Skipstead S. *Sacro occipital technique seminar*, Omaha, Nebraska, October, 2003.

Burnier A. The side effects of the chiropractic adjustment. *Chiropr Pediatr* 1995; 1: 22–24.

Cohen E. Case history; an eight year old asthma patient. *Todays Chiropr* 1988; 17: 81.

DeJarnette MB. *Cranial Technique*. Private publication, Nebraska City, Nebraska, 1979.

Garde R. Asthma and chiropractic. *Chiropr Pediatr* 1994; 1: 9–16.

Hodge L, Salome CM, Peat JK, Haby MM, Xuan W, Woodcock AJ. Consumption of oily fish and childhood asthma risk. *Med J Aust* 1996; 164: 137–140.

Lau BH, Riesen SK, Truong KP, Lau EW, Rohdewald P, Barreta RA. Pycnogenol as an adjunct in the management of childhood asthma. *J Asthma* 2004; 41: 825–832.

Mega JJ. Bronchial asthma. *Am Chiropr* 1982; 66: 26–27.

Nielsen NH, Brontfort G, Bendix T, Madsen F, Weeke B. Chronic asthma and chiropractic spinal manipulation: a randomized clinical trial. *Clin Exp Allergy* 1995; 25: 80–88.

Rubin RN, Navon L, Cassano PA. Relationship of serum antioxidants to asthma prevalence in youth. *Am J Resp Crit Care Med* 2004; 169: 393–398.

Saxon A, Decamp ON. *Sacro Occipital Technique Cranial Participant Guide, 3rd edn.* Prairie Village, Kansas: Sacro Occipital Resource International, 1990.

Schmidt MA. *Healing Childhood Ear Infections.* Berkley, California: North Atlantic Books, 1996.

Tepas EC, Umetsu DT. Immunology and allergy. In *Nelson's Essentials of Pediatrics*, Berhman RE, Kliegman RE (eds). Philadelphia: WB Saunders, 2002.

Cerebral palsy

Arbuckle BE. *The Collected Writings of Beryl E Arbuckle.* Indianapolis: American Academy of Osteopathy, 1994.

Carreiro JE. *An Osteopathic Approach to Children.* Edinburgh: Churchill Livingstone, 2003.

Collins KF et al. The efficacy of upper cervical chiropractic care on children and adults with cerebral palsy: a preliminary report. *Chiropr Pediatr* 1994; 1: 13–15.

Fitzgerald M, Styles E. Osteopathic hospitals solution to DRG's may be OMT. *DO* 1984: 97–101.

Golden LM, Van Egmond CA. Longitudinal clinical case study: multi-disciplinary care of a child with multiple functional and developmental disorders. In *Proceedings of the National Conference on Chiropractic and Pediatrics*, 1992, pp 24–39.

Kuban K, Leviton A. Cerebral palsy. *N Engl J Med* 1990; 330: 188–195.

Laisram N, Srivastava VK, Srivastava RK. Cerebral palsy – an etiologic study. *Ind J Pediatr* 1992; 59: 723–728.

Lohse-Busch H. Therapy with manual medicine and physiotherapy applied to children with cerebral palsy. *J Orthop Med* 2003; 25: 22–23.

Lohse-Busch H, Riedel M, Falland R, Sailer-Kramer B, Reime U, Kraemer M. Combined treatment with techniques of manual medicine and physiotherapy in children with infantile cerebral palsy. *Man Med* 2003; 41: 279–287.

McCoy M, Malakhova E, Safronov Y. Improvement in paraspinal muscle tone, autonomic function and quality of life in four children with cerebral palsy undergoing subluxation based chiropractic care: four retrospective case studies. *J Vert Sublux Reas* 2000; 4.

McMullen M. Chiropractic and the handicapped child. Part II. Cerebral palsy. *ICA Rev Chiropr* 1990; 46: 39, 41–43.

Rosenbloom L. Diagnosis and management of cerebral palsy. *Arch Dis Child* 1995; 72: 350–354.

Sulkes SB, Dosa NP. Developmental and behavioural pediatrics. In *Nelson's Essentials of Pediatrics*, Behrman RE, Kliegman RM (eds). Philadelphia: WB Saunders, 2002.

Sweat RW, Ammons DL. Case study: the treatment of a cerebral palsy patient. *Todays Chiropr* 1988; 17: 51–52.

Webster LL. Case study: mental retardation/cerebral palsy. *Chiropr Pediatr* 1994; 1: 15–16.

Common paediatric syndromes

Illustrations in Chapter Eight

Chapter 9

Attention deficit hyperactivity disorder, dyslexia and dyspraxia

ATTENTION DEFICIT HYPERACTIVITY DISORDER

Attention deficit hyperactivity disorder (ADHD) covers a broad spectrum of behavioural disorders. The child may be particularly hyperactive or predominately inattentive, or may strongly exhibit both characteristics. The diagnosis is a clinical one and, in the UK, is made on the basis of the World Health Organization (1992) classification, including hyperactivity as a key criterion.

Current medical treatment in the UK and most other Western countries focuses on using methylphenidate (Ritalin) and dextroamphetamine (Dextrostat). My experience is that children on these products respond less well to chiropractic intervention so it may be worth initiating chiropractic care during the school holidays as many children are, owing to their previous disruptive behaviour, allowed to attend school only if they take these drugs. It is worth discussing the idea of a 'drug break' with the parents, school and general practitioner.

Goddard, in her book *Reflexes, Learning and Behavior* (2002), discusses how primitive or neonatal reflex retention may play a role in ADHD, dyslexia and dyspraxia. These reflexes should be inhibited by the development of adult postural and startle reflexes, but when this inhibition fails, the child may be left with physical and psychological consequences. In practice, I have found that children diagnosed within the ADHD spectrum will often show some degree of primitive reflex retention, especially the Moro reflex. The long-term effects of a retained Moro reflex can include (adapted with permission from Goddard 2002):

- vestibular disorders: motion sickness, poor balance and coordination;
- physical timidity;
- visual perceptual problems, such as a stimulus-bound effect (an inability to ignore extraneous and irrelevant visual material, e.g. movements in the visual periphery);
- slow pupillary reactions, photosensitivity, and difficulty with print on white paper and reactions to fluorescent lighting;
- auditory hypersensitivity: difficulty in 'screening out' extraneous noise;
- allergies, decreased immunity and recurrent infections;
- adverse drug reactions;
- easily fatigued;
- dislike of change;
- poorly developed carbon dioxide reflex;
- reactive hypoglycaemia.

Possible secondary psychological symptoms include:

- anxiety;
- an excessive reaction to stimuli: mood swings, tense muscle tone, inability to accept criticism;
- cycles of hyperactivity followed by fatigue;
- difficulty in making decisions;
- low self-esteem and insecurity.

It has been my experience that some babies show a hyperactive Moro response. These are infants who startle very easily with noise, movement or touch, and cry readily. The parents have to 'tiptoe' around the house and move the infant cautiously to avoid the baby jumping and crying. The primary finding that these infants have in common appears to be severe sphenoid bone restriction. It is possible that these babies will grow up and form at least a proportion of those children diagnosed with ADHD.

Imagine a child 7 years old with retention of the Moro reflex. There is background noise in the classroom, and the movements of other children invade his peripheral vision. He cannot screen out these stimuli and concentration lapses. The child is tired and irritable, with low adrenal function resulting from chronic hyperstimulation and reactive hypoglycaemia. He has a chocolate bar in the mid-morning break, the sugar 'hit' powers him up again, and he bounces off the classroom walls.

This may be an oversimplistic picture, with many more contributory genetic and psychosocial factors, but it can play a significant part in the process.

Moro reflex retention tests

These tests are primarily applicable to children over 5 years of age: younger than this, children may well have difficulty in performing them accurately.

Standing test

The child is instructed to stand with her arms out in front, with her elbows slightly bent and her palms inwards as if forming a circle; her head is tilted backwards looking at the ceiling. The child is then asked to sway backwards on to her heels and deliberately overbalance backwards. Prior to this manoeuvre, the doctor instructs the child to clasp her arms rapidly around her chest as she feels herself begin to overbalance backwards. The doctor stands behind the child to catch her as she falls. It is necessary to reassure the child that she will not fall to the ground but will be caught (Figure 9.1).

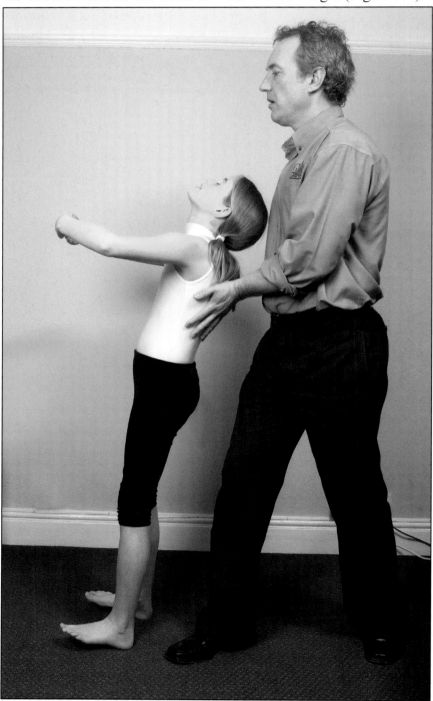

Figure 9.1 Persistent Moro test – standing.

Supine test

This is good for older children who tend to be less trusting about being caught as they overbalance. The child lies supine with the arms in the same position as in the standing test. She needs to have her head and neck in free space off the bench as a degree of cervical hyperextension is necessary (Figure 9.2a). The doctor holds the child's head in a neutral position and tells her to clasp her hands across her chest rapidly as her head is allowed to drop down a few inches (Figure 9.2b). It is necessary to take care to gain the child's confidence in order to ensure success with this test.

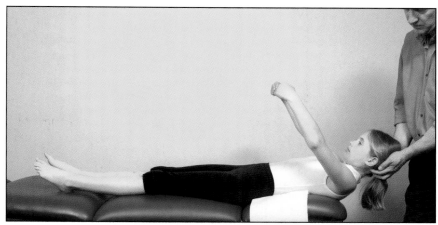
Figure 9.2a Persistent Moro test – supine start.

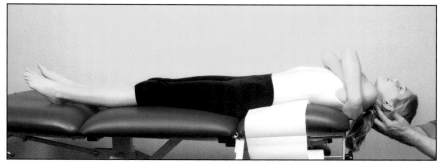
Figure 9.2b Persistant Moro test – supine finish..

Results

A rapid and complete adduction of the arms across the chest at the completion of the tests indicates no likelihood of Moro reflex retention. Any degree of initial abduction of the arms or hesitation in movement may, however, indicate some degree of Moro reflex retention.

Treatment of ADHD

Soft tissues

Release and balancing of the transverse fascial planes of the diaphragm and pelvic floor is important. Adrenal inhibition in children demonstrating high levels of hyperactivity is useful. This is accomplished by holding pressure over the adrenal glands anteriorly with the thumb and fingers of one hand while holding a simultaneous pressure on the T9 transverse processes (Figure 9.3). Full adrenal and pancreatic chiropractic manipulative reflex technique protocols can also be used (Bathie 2000).

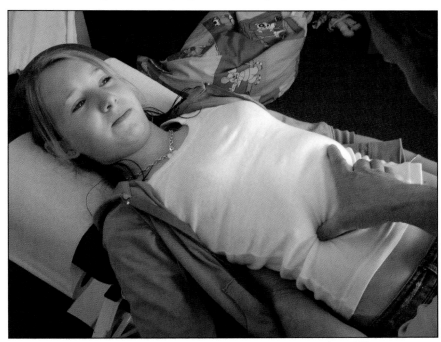
Figure 9.3 Adrenal inhibition – pressure is held over the adrenal glands and T9 transverse processes.

Spine

Check the function of the upper cervical vertebrae, T8–T9 and the thoraco-lumbar junction; be cautious, however, not to carry out too much adjustment on one visit as this can occasionally aggravate the condition via over stimulation.

Cranium

It is essential to establish normal sphenoid motion. To do this, it is often also necessary to address the occiput and frontal bones (Chapter 6). Cranial rhythmic impulse balancing often helps to slow the cranial rhythm, which can in turn help to decrease hyperactivity.

The doctor takes a vault contact on the child with the index fingers to the frontal bones, the third fingers to the sphenoid wings, the ring fingers to the squamous suture, the little fingers to the occipitomastoid suture and the thumbs to the parietal bones. The cranial pulses are then balanced by using gentle pressure from the side of greatest pulsation towards that of least pulsation until all are balanced (Figure 9.4; Saxon and Decamp 1990).

Diet

A number of authors have proposed dietary treatment for ADHD (Feingold 1975, Crook 1991), with some success reported by parents. Feingold (1975) recommended avoiding natural salicylates, food colourings and preservatives. In my experience, the avoidance of food colourings and preservatives is desirable, but the primary dietary consideration is an avoidance of sugar. Refined sugar tends to perpetuate the swings of blood sugar from which so many ADHD children suffer. I recommend that the whole family should follow this avoidance regime or it will feel to the child that he or she is yet again being punished, which will negatively affect their often already low self-esteem.

Supplementation

In my practice, I use a hair analysis for toxic elements and mineral levels on all children with ADHD, often finding high levels of lead, mercury, antimony and aluminum in the hair. Common mineral deficiencies also identified include those of zinc, magnesium and chromium. Supplementation can then be tailored to a removal of the toxic elements (most companies undertaking hair analysis will recommend a protocol) and supplementing the specific deficiencies.

A growing number of studies show that multivitamin and mineral supplements combined with fish oil help some aggressive and antisocial behaviour patterns and developmental coordination disorders, as well as non-verbal learning, although not specifically ADHD (Schoenthaler et al 2000, Benton 2001,Gesch et al 2002). I therefore tend to recommend a broad-spectrum multivitamin and

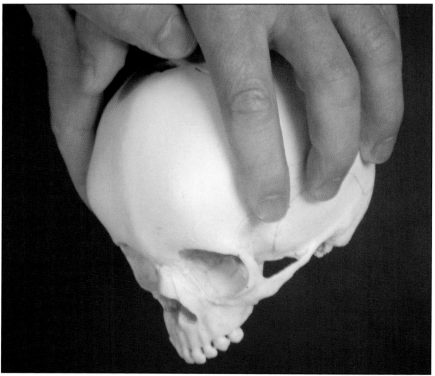

Figure 9.4   Cranial rhythmic impulse balancing. Note the finger contacts to the frontal, sphenoid, temporal and parietal bones, and occiput.

mineral supplement with at least two capsules of fish oil per day.

Low iron levels have been identified as occurring more commonly in children with ADHD (Konofal et al 2004). Zinc and magnesium supplementation has also been shown to be helpful (Kozielec and Starobrat-Hermelin 1997, Starobrat-Hermelin and Kozeilec 1997, Bilici et al 2004). Zinc, iron and magnesium all have some positive effects when used as supplements, but I would prefer to give additional mineral supplementation with the broad-spectrum multivitamin–mineral supplement only when low levels of the relevant elements are shown up on hair analysis.

Exercise

Sea anemone exercise. The sea anemone exercise specifically inhibits the Moro reflex (Goddard 2002). The child lies supine and adopts a position of neck, arm and leg flexion with the arms and legs crossed. Very slowly, the child unwinds from this position to about half way and then closes down again slowly to the flexed position. This should take 5–8 seconds for one cycle (Figure 9.5a, 9.5b and 9.5c). This exercise should be repeated eight times once per day until the persistent Moro reflex is inhibited.

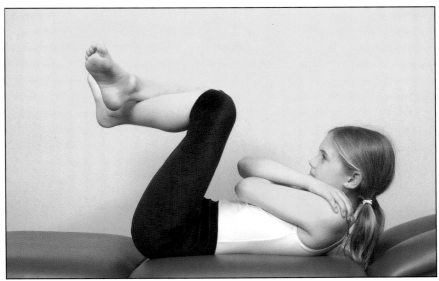

Figure 9.5a The sea anemone exercise start.

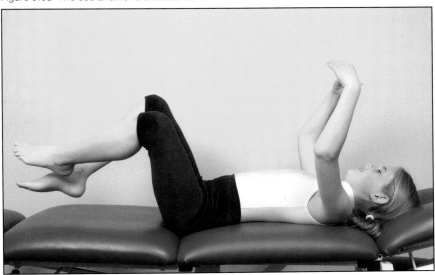

Figure 9.5b The sea anemone exercise middle.

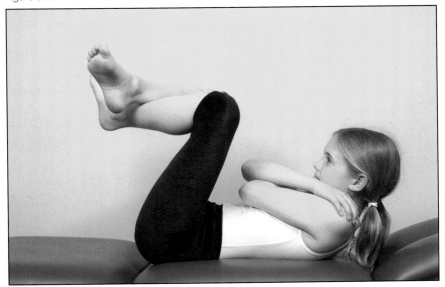

Figure 9.5c The sea anemone exercise finish.

DYSLEXIA AND DYSPRAXIA

These two conditions are presented together as there is often an overlap between them, 80% of children diagnosed with dyslexia having some symptoms of dyspraxia, and up to 80% of children with a diagnosis of dyspraxia having some symptoms of dyslexia (Goddard 2002). Indeed, ADHD might also have been included here as this too shows a considerable overlap. The assessment protocols discussed later in this chapter are applicable to both conditions and attempt to identify the 'broken links' in the individual child's neurological make up. The treatment strategies focus on trying to repair these broken links. The test and treatment protocols to be discussed are relevant to any child showing low-grade symptoms of slowed or delayed development or poor coordination, language or writing skills.

It is important to have accurately recorded test protocol results so that changes in the child's condition can be assessed by the chiropractor somewhat objectively rather than simply by whether the teacher or the parent thinks that there has been progress. Remember that parents *want* to see change so they may not be the most reliable guides to the child's progress. I suggest that re assessments of the test protocols

be made every five or six treatments. It is also my experience that if a child suffering from dyslexia/dyspraxia is going to respond to chiropractic care, which certainly appears to be the norm, improvements will be noted within five visits.

Test protocol

Primitive reflexes

Goddard (2002) noted that there will often be a cluster of abnormal primitive and postural reflexes in children with dyslexia and or dyspraxia so it is useful to test for their presence. The reflexes can be scored using a 5-point scale ranging from 0 to 4 inclusive. A score of zero means that no abnormality is present, whereas a score of 4 denotes a major retention of the reflexes. It takes some experience in using the tests to score them satisfactorily, but, although somewhat subjective, these are a useful tool.

Most children will show traces of abnormality in one or two of the reflexes and can compensate for these, but a cluster of abnormal reflexes can adversely affect motor development and neonatal skills.

Moro reflex. This is described in the section on ADHD above.

Palmar grasp reflex. The grasp reflex emerges in utero, is fully present at birth and is generally inhibited by about 3 months of

age. It is possibly a continuation of reflexes needed earlier in human evolution, when it was necessary for the young to cling to their mother for safety. The reflex can be elicited by sucking movements, and the action of sucking may cause hand-kneading movements in time with the suck (the Babkin response).

The effects of palmar grasp retention (Goddard 2002) are:

- poor manual dexterity;
- the lack of a 'pincer' grip so the child is unable to grip a pencil properly when writing;
- speech difficulties – from a persistent relationship between hand and mouth movements via the Babkin response, which hinders the development of muscle control at the front of the mouth and can affect articulation;
- a palm that may be hypersensitive to touch;
- the child making mouth movements when writing.

To test for palmar grasp retention, the child's hand is fully opened (flat) and is very gently stroked across the palm (Figure 9.6). Withdrawal or closure of the hand indicates a retention of the grasp reflex, whereas a flicker of movement of the thumb or fingers indicates a lesser degree of retention.

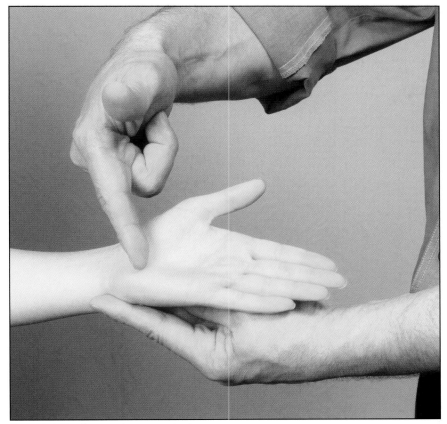

Figure 9.6 Persistent palmar grasp test.

The effects of asymmetric tonic neck reflex retention (Goddard 2002) are:

- poor balance;
- homolateral movements and lack of a cross-crawl pattern;
- difficulty crossing the midline or manipulating an object with both hands;
- poor ocular pursuit, particularly when following an object at the midline;
- mixed laterality of the hand, eye, ear and foot;
- poor handwriting and expression of ideas on paper;
- visual perceptual difficulties; particularly with the symmetrical representation of figures.

Asymmetrical tonic neck reflex. The asymmetrical tonic neck reflex emerges in utero and is fully present at birth; indeed, it is thought to aid in the birth process by lowering the shoulder when the head undergoes internal rotation. This reflex helps to ensure a free passage of air if the baby is prone and the development of extensor tone. If retained, it will inhibit a fluent cross-crawl pattern when crawling and make the manipulation of objects with both hands difficult.

Retention of this reflex can be tested for as follows. The child kneels on all fours with the arms straight and is asked to very slowly to turn her head all the way to one side (full range of motion) and then slowly all the way to the other side (Figure 9.7). This is repeated five times. A strong degree of reflex retention is indicated by one arm giving way and the body dipping down to the bench. A much lesser degree of retention is indicated by just a slight bend of one elbow.

Tonic labyrinthine reflex. The tonic labyrinthine reflex (TLR) is a two-part reflex, the TLR forwards emerging in utero with body flexion occurring as the

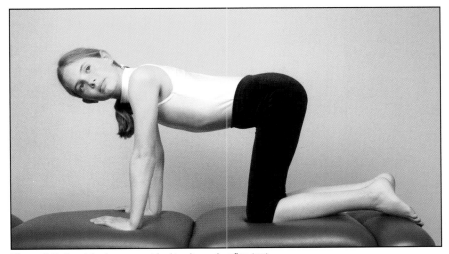

Figure 9.7 Persistent asymmetrical tonic neck reflex test.

133

Dyslexia and dyspraxia

neck is flexed. It is inhibited by about 4 months of age. The TLR backwards emerges at birth and is inhibited in a gradual progression from about 5 months to 3 years old. The TLR and Moro reflexes are closely linked in early life, both are vestibular in origin, and both are activated by labyrinthine stimulation via head movement and alteration of position. The TLR is involved in the infant's reaction to gravity and the development of body tone.

The effects of a TLR forwards retention (Goddard 2002) are:

- a stooped posture;
- hypotonic muscles;
- poor balance;
- motion sickness;
- being poor at games;
- oculomotor dysfunction – difficulties with visual perception and spatial awareness;
- poor sequencing.

The effects of a TLR backwards retention are:

- walking on the toes;
- hypertonic muscles, especially extensors;
- poor balance and coordination;
- motion sickness;
- oculomotor dysfunction – difficulties with visual perception and spatial awareness;
- poor sequencing skills.

In the test for the TLR, the child stands with the feet together and the arms straight down by the sides of the body and is asked to tilt her head back into full extension and close her eyes (the doctor should stand behind the child in case of loss of balance; Figure 9.8a). After a count of 10, ask the child to flex her neck fully and look at her toes for a further count of 10 (Figure 9.8b).

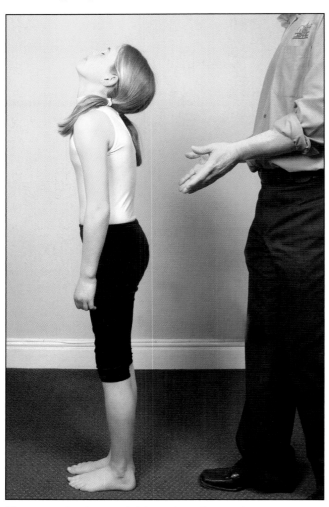

Figure 9.8a Persistent tonic labyrinthine reflex test: backwards.

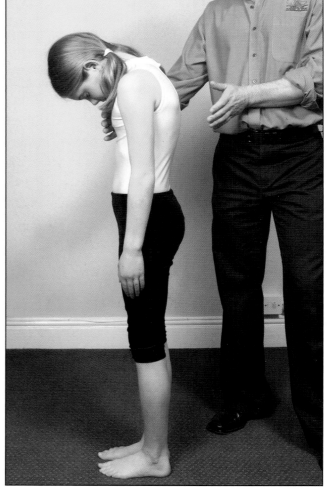

Figure 9.8b Persistent tonic labyrinthine reflex test: forwards.

134

Repeat this 10 times. A child with a retained reflex will tend to show a loss of balance, and a significant change in muscle tone, dizziness and nausea may also be encountered. A mildly retained reflex will show a slight alteration in balance, possibly with the toes flexing to hold balance.

Symmetrical tonic neck reflex. The reflex emerges at 6–9 months of age and is inhibited by 9–11 months old. It is present for only a short period of time and enables the child to assume a crawling position.

The effects of the symmetrical tonic neck reflex retention are:

- poor posture;
- a slumped sitting position;
- a simian (ape-like) walk;
- a 'w' leg position when sitting on the floor;
- poor hand–eye coordination;
- difficulties with the readjustment of binocular vision, for example from blackboard to desk;
- slowness at copying tasks;
- difficulty learning to swim;
- poor attention when having to sit still.

In the symmetrical tonic neck reflex test, the child kneels on all fours and is asked to slowly flex her neck and look back between her legs for 5 seconds (Figure 9.9a). She is then asked to slowly extend her neck to look at the ceiling, with her arms straight and her body still; this position is held for 5 seconds (Figure 9.9b). This can be repeated six times. A strongly retained reflex is indicated by a bending of the arms to the floor and a movement of the hips back on to the ankles. A slightly retained reflex is indicated by slight elbow flexion or hip movement.

Other tests

The following tests are tests of balance, coordination and left and right hemispheric integration, and are aimed for use on a child of approximately 7 years of age. An allowance for the expected lower level of brain development must be made if these are used for testing younger children.

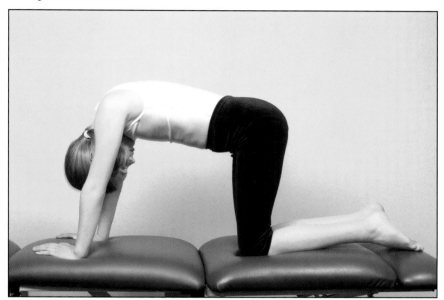

Figure 9.9a Persistent symmetrical tonic neck reflex test part 1.

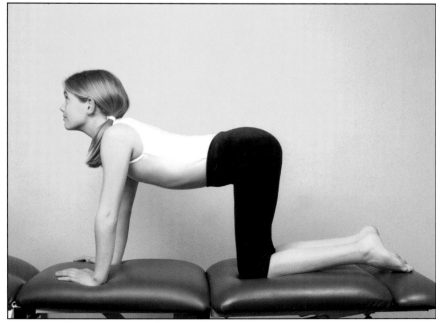

Figure 9.9b Persistent symmetrical tonic neck reflex test part 2.

135

Dyslexia and dyspraxia

Tandem walk. The child is asked to walk slowly heel to toe looking straight ahead. This is then performed backwards and then repeated with the eyes shut (Figure 9.10). Shutting the eyes creates a much stronger test of the labyrinthine mechanisms and might well prove to be a problem for the chiropractor too! For ease of recording and reassessment, this test can be given a numeral score, as with the primitive reflexes.

Frog walk. The child is asked to walk slowly on the outsides of her feet, taking small steps. This is again done forwards, the backwards, then repeated with the eyes shut (Figure 9.11).

Many children will show poor balance with their eyes shut.

Synkinesis. This is evaluated by getting the child to perform a repetitive action with only one hand while the other is immobile. Children should be capable of this after 8 years of age. An inability to do this has been linked to learning and

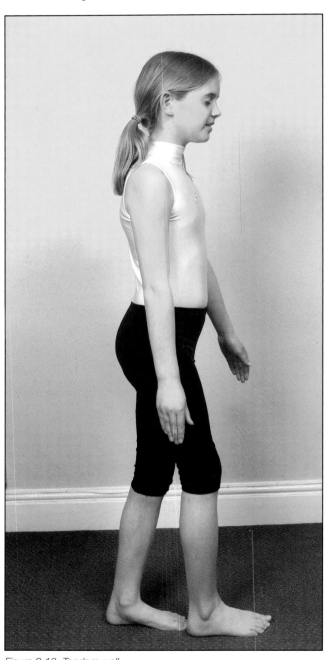

Figure 9.10 Tandem walk.

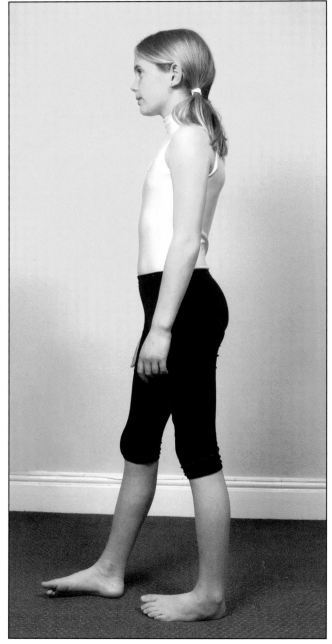

Figure 9.11 Frog walk.

behavioural dysfunction (Levine et al 1983).

Dysdiadochokinesis. The child is asked to pronate and supinate both hands simultaneously (Figure 9.12). Incoordination or an inability to perform the test implies a degree of developmental immaturity (Levine et al 1983).

Stimulus extinction. The child is asked to shut her eyes and is then touched simultaneously on her hand and face (Figure 9.13). After 7 years of age, children should be able to identify not just the proximal, but also the distal point of touch. Failure to do so is an indicator of developmental dysfunction or immaturity (Levine et al 1983).

Choreiform movements. The child is asked to stand with her arms straight out in front, fingers spread and mouth open with the tongue stuck out for 30 seconds (Figure 9.14). Choreiform movement identified in the fingers of children over 5 years of age may be associated with hyperactivity, behavioural problems and learning difficulties (Levine et al 1983).

Left–right discrimination. By 6 years of age, the child should be able to follow a command to touch her left ear. By 8 years of age, the child should be able to follow a command to touch her left ear with her right hand, reaching across the midline. By 10 years of age, she should

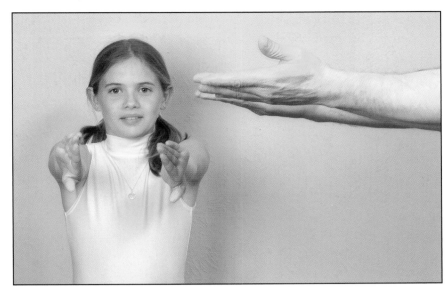

Figure 9.12 Dysdiadochokinesis.

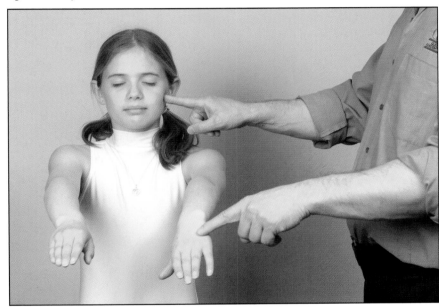

Figure 9.13 Stimulus extinction.

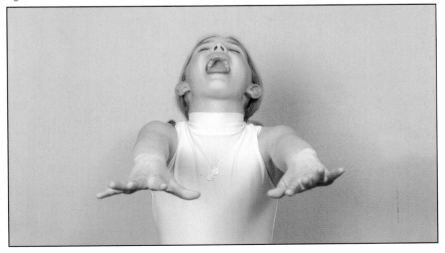

Figure 9.14 Choreiform movement test.

Dyslexia and dyspraxia

be able to march on the spot in a smooth cross-crawl pattern (Davies 2000). When over 10 years of age, children should be able to identify left and right on the examiner when facing him (Figure 9.15).

Hemispheric motor integration. The child lies supine, the arm on one side and the contralateral leg being raised to 40 degrees. The child is then asked to resist a downward pressure on both limbs at the same time (Figure 9.16). The test is then repeated with the other arm and leg. Weakening of the contralateral arm or leg, or both, indicates some degree of failure of hemispheric motor integration and should be recorded.

Hemispheric motor integration across the midline can be tested as above but this time with the limbs crossed over the midline of the body (Figure 9.17). Again any weakness should be recorded. Clinically, I have found that those children who exhibit a retained asymmetrical tonic neck reflex often show weakness across the midline.

Eye-tracking. Two tests can be employed for eye-tracking.

In the *static* test, eye-tracking is tested as in a cranial nerve examination, with the addition of testing a strong indicator muscle in concert with each eye position. I use a general shoulder flexion test (at about 70

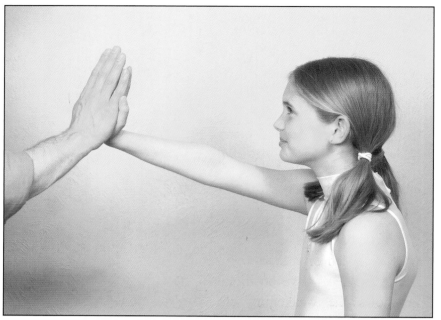
Figure 9.15 Left–right discrimination in an 11-year-old.

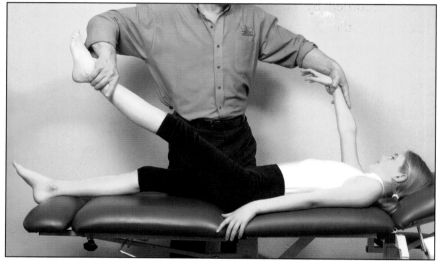
Figure 9.16 Hemispheric motor integration test.

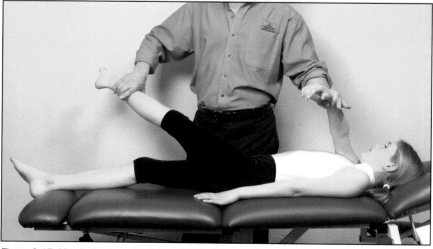
Figure 9.17 Hemispheric motor integration test across the midline.

138

degrees) while supine. Each eye position is challenged (the child being asked to gaze at a brightly coloured pen) with the muscle test, and any weakness is recorded (Figure 9.18). Any weakness elicited is often associated with the individual child's problems, for example difficulty catching a ball – weakness on superior gaze, difficulty on reading – weakness on inferior gaze. The results can be recorded on a star chart (Figure 9.19). Any eye position that shows the weakening of a previously strong muscle can be recorded by circling or underlining the X relevant to that eye position.

In the *dynamic* test, the eyes are taken through a left-to-right and up-and-down dynamic movement pattern. They are observed for jumping, loss of tracking, blinking or weakness of a strong indicator muscle, all of which indicate difficulty with tracking. A figure-of-8 pattern is then followed, and the child is observed as above.

Recording test results

Table 9.1 (see page 146) provides a grid for recording the results of the above examinations.

Treatment of Dyslexia and Dyspraxia

The assessment identifies the areas of the child's neurological dysfunction, revealing the areas in which there is a lack of linkage or improper integration of the

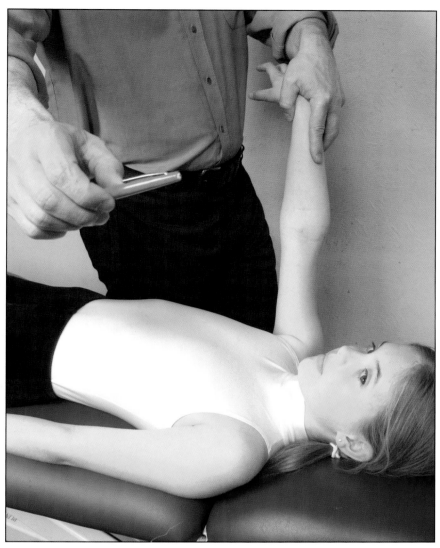

Figure 9.18 Eye-tracking test.

Superior right gaze	X	X	X	
	X	X	X	
	X	X	X	Inferior left gaze

Figure 9.19 Star chart for the static eye-tracking test.

neurological system. This may be related to the vestibular reflexes, postural reflexes, eye-tracking, hemispheric integration or general neurological immaturity. Treatment is focused on these incomplete neurological links in order to allow the nervous system

to catch up on its development.

The areas to concentrate on in the initial phase of care are the static eye positions, hemispheric integration and hemispheric integration across the midline. It is important as a first step, however, to try to ameliorate any of the chronic postural patterns that the child shows. This is done by balancing the transverse fascial planes (psoas release, diaphragm release and pelvic floor balancing) and correcting the pelvis, sacrum and upper cervical vertebrae. This may mean, in an individual child with significant subluxation patterns in these areas, that it takes one or two treatment sessions to get the child into condition and therefore allow work to begin on his or her specific dyslexic/dyspraxic patterns. It is particularly important that the pelvis is stable prior to this so supine blocking is utilised when indicated.

Stimulation of the oculomotor reflex via the pupillary light reflex is used while the greater wings of the sphenoid are taken into flexion (Figure 9.20). This causes a bombardment of, among other structures, the red nucleus and the reticular formation, which affects eye coordination, limb muscle tone and the fight and flight response.

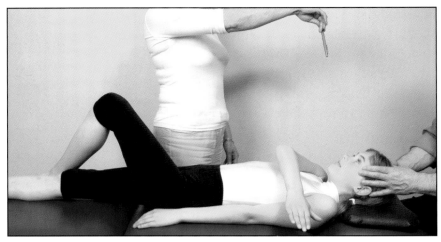

Figure 9.20 Treatment for dyslexia/dyspraxia – sphenoid release with correction of eye-tracking and hemispheric integration across the midline.

Treatment summary

1. Level the transverse fascial planes:
   - psoas/diaphragm;
   - pelvic floor;
   - thoracic outlet.
2. Spinal correction, including the sacrum and upper cervical vertebrae.
3. Stabilise any pelvic instability with supine blocks.
4. Release any restricted cranial sutures; this stimulates type I and II mechanoreceptors in the cranial sutures.

5. Take the greater wings of the sphenoid very gently into flexion (downwards and forward) while the eyes and body are in the position that elicited skeletal weakness as found in the test protocols. A pen torch is then used to stimulate a rapid pupillary contraction. If the body position involved a weakness of the opposite arm and leg, the child should be instructed to wiggle the fingers and toes of the limbs that showed the weakness as this will help the correction.

For example, in a child with a grade 2 retention of the asymmetrical tonic neck reflex and TLR, the following might be found:

- Tandem walk grade 3 and frog walk grade 3.
- Left arm and right leg weak across the midline.
- Eye-tracking, dynamic 3.
- Eye-tracking, static

X	Ⓧ	X
X	X	X
X	X	X

Treatment is then be carried out as follows. After correction of the fascial planes, spine, sacrum, pelvis and cranial sutures, the child is positioned with the left arm across the midline wiggling the fingers, the right leg across the midline wiggling the toes, and the eyes tracked up to a superior gaze as the sphenoid is released into flexion (i.e. simultaneously bringing the greater wings of the sphenoid gently antero-inferiorly). A pen torch is then shone in the eyes to elicit a pupillary contraction. This sets the correction, and the child should then be asked to walk around the room. A reassessment is then performed to see which of the original findings the adjustment has affected. This methodology can then be used for any remaining problems with eye-tracking or other areas of dysfunction that can be identified.

Once left–right brain hemisphere integration has been established and the static eye-tracking tests are strong, dynamic eye-tracking should be addressed using the same principle of using the pupillary light reflex and sphenoid release into flexion while the child is following the movement of a pen torch in a figure-of-8.

Any other areas showing dysfunction can be addressed in the same way: find the task the child finds challenging and while he or she is doing the task, for example repeating a sequence of numbers, take the greater wings of the sphenoid into flexion and activate the oculomotor nucleus via the pupillary light reflex. Each area of dysfunction will usually require one or two applications of this technique. Do not address more than one or two areas with each treatment as the central nervous system needs time to adapt to the new linkages that have been made. Exercises related to the area of dysfunction, for example eye-tracking, cross-crawl or sequencing numbers or words, are useful to ensure proper integration.

An evaluation of progress should be performed after the fifth and tenth visits, re checking the scores on the entire range of test protocols. If there is still a significant cluster or retained reflexes are present with little diminution in their scores, a reflex inhibition exercise programme needs to be undertaken with an appropriately trained individual. Most children will, however, have made significant progress, and future treatment should be focused on any remaining areas of dysfunction.

Diet

A diet low in refined sugars, artificial colourings and additives is recommended as this tends to help the concentration level. If food sensitivities are suspected, these should be tested for and eliminated if necessary.

Supplementation

Essential fatty acids have commonly been shown to be deficient in children with dyslexia and may even predict the degree of reading difficulty (Richardson et al 2000). Supplementation has also been shown to be effective in children with learning difficulties (Richardson and Puri 2002, Richardson and Montgomery 2005). A good quality multivitamin and mineral supplement is also recommended, as is a hair analysis and the specific supplementation of any deficiencies noted.

Exercises

1   Eye tracking exercises are very useful and should be given to all children exhibiting eye tracking problems. The easiest way is to ask the parents to move a brightly coloured object slowly and steadily in the same pattern used to check the child's tracking and get them to follow it with their eyes only. This makes a star shape and should be performed 5-8 times twice per day.

2   For those children with coordination problems and/or weak-

ness on the hemispheric integration tests, cross crawl type exercise are useful. I usually get them to march on the spot with a high contra lateral knee and arm lift for 30 repetitions twice per day. If they change to a homo lateral pattern during the repetitions they must stop and start from the beginning again. For some severely compromised individuals it can be necessary for the parents to perform the exercises on the child initially, (moving opposite arms and legs) with the child lying supine.

3   For children with vestibular problems an exercise known as windmills (Goddard 2002) is of great use. The standing child with arms out laterally at 90 degrees rotates slowly 360 degrees, and then stands still with eyes shut, with their arms down for a count of 10; this is then repeated in the other direction. The whole exercise is repeated 3 times in both directions. The parents should observe them for any unsteadiness, once the child is able to perform the task without a wobble, they do 2 and then 3 circuits in each direction, always with the eyes shut for a count of 10 between. It can take weeks or months to get up to three circuits but by then the child's balance should be improved, as will any tendency towards motion sickness.

REFERENCES

Attention deficit hyperactivity disorder

Bathie R. *Chiropractic Manipulative Reflex Technique Manual*. Prairie Village, Kansas: Sacro Occipital Resource International, 2000.

Benton D. Micronutrient supplementation and the intelligence of children. *Neurosci Behav Dev* 2001; 25: 297–309.

Bilici M, Yildirim F, Kandil S, Bekaroglu M, Yilidirmis S, Deger O, Ulgen M, Yildiran A, Askau H. Double blind placebo controlled study of zinc sulphate in the treatment of attention deficit hyperactivity disorder. *Prog Neuropsycopharmacol Biol Psychiatry* 2004; 28: 181–190.

Crook WG. *Help for the Hyperactive Child*. Jackson, Tennessee: Professional Books, 1991.

Fiengold B. *Why Is your Child Hyperactive?* New York: Random House, 1975.

Gesch CB, Hammond SM, Hampson SE, Eves A, Crowder MJ. Influence of supplementary vitamins, minerals and essential fatty acids on the antisocial behavior of young adult prisoners. Randomised placebo-controlled trial. *Br J Psychiatry* 2002; 181: 22–28.

Goddard S. *Reflexes, Learning and Behavior a window into the child's mind*. Eugene, Oregon: Fern Ridge Press, 2002.

Konofal E, Lecendreum M, Arnuf I, Maren MC. Iron deficiency in children with attention deficit hyperactivity disorder. *Arch Pediatr Adolesc Med* 2004; 158: 1113–1115.

Kozielec T, Starobrat-Hermelin B. Assessment of magnesium levels in children with attention deficit hyperactivity disorder (ADHD). *Magnes Res* 1997; 10: 142–148.

Saxon A, Decamp ON. *SOT Cranial Participant Guide, 3rd edn*. Prairie Village Kansas: Sacro Occipital Resource International, 1990.

Scheonthaler SJ, Bier JD. The effect of vitamin–mineral supplementation on juvenile delinquency among American school age children: a randomized double blind placebo controlled trial. *J Altern Complement Med* 2000; 6: 7–17.

Starobrat-Hermelin B, Kozeilec T. The effects of magnesium physiological supplementation on hyperactivity in children with attention deficit hyperactivity disorder (ADHD). Positive response to magnesium oral loading test. *Magnes Res* 1997; 10: 149–156.

World Health Organization. ICD 10 Classification of Mental and Behavioral Disorders: *Clinical Descriptions and Diagnostic Guidelines*. Geneva: WHO, 1992.

Dyslexia/dyspraxia

Davies NJ. Developmental assessment, neuromaturational delay and school learning difficulties. *In Chiropractic Pediatrics*, Davies NJ (ed.). Edinburgh: Churchill Livingstone, 2000, pp 121–136.

Goddard S. *Reflexes, Learning and Behavior a window into the child's mind*. Eugene, Oregon: Fern Ridge Press, 2002.

Levine MD, Carey WB, Crocker AV, Gross RT. *Developmental Behavioral Pediatrics*. Philadelphia: WB Saunders, 1983.

Richardson AJ, Puri BK. A randomised double blind placebo controlled study of the effects of supplementation with highly unsaturated fatty acids on ADHD related symptoms in children with specific learning difficulties. *Prog Neuropsychopharm Biol Psychiatry* 2002; 26: 233–239.

Richardson AJ, Calvin CM, Clisby C, Scheonheimer DR, Montgomery P, Hall JA, Hebb G, Westwood E, Talcott JB, Stein JF. Fatty acid deficiency signs predict the severity of reading and related deficiencies in dyslexic children. *Prostaglandins Leukotr Essent Fatty Acids* 2000; 63: 69–74.

Richardson AJ, Montgomery P. The Oxford–Durham study: a randomized controlled trial of dietary supplementation with fatty acids in children with developmental coordination disorder. *Pediatrics* 2005; 115: 1360–1366.

Illustrations in Chapter Nine

Dyslexia and dyspraxia

Recording test results					
Reflexes	0	1	2	3	4
Moro					
Palmar					
Asymmetrical tonic neck reflex					
Tonic labyrinthine reflex					
Symmetrical tonic neck reflex					
Other tests					
Tandem walk					
Frog walk					
Synkinesis					
Dysdiadochokinesis					
Stimulus extinction					
Choreiform movement					
Left–right discrimination					
Cross-crawl standing					
Hemispheric integration					
Hemispheric integration across the midline					
Eye-tracking –dynamic					
Eye-tracking – static X X X X X X X X X					

Table 9.1 Table for recording test results

Index